12

Spinal Angiomas

With contributions by

Valentine Logue
FRCP, FRCS
Professor of Neurosurgery
in the Institute of
Neurology
University of London

B. E. Kendall
FRCP, FFR
Consultant Radiologist
National Hospitals for
Nervous Diseases and
the Middlesex Hospital

M.J. Aminoff
BSc, MD, MRCP
Senior Registrar,
National Hospitals for
Nervous Diseases,
London

Spinal Angiomas

Blackwell Scientific
Publications
OXFORD LONDON
EDINBURGH MELBOURNE

© 1976 Blackwell Scientific
Publications,
Osney Mead, Oxford,
8 John Street, London WC1,
9 Forrest Road, Edinburgh,
PO Box 9, North Balwyn,
Victoria, Australia.

ISBN 0 632 00237 9

First published 1976

Distributed in the
United States of America by
J. B. Lippincott Company,
Philadelphia,
and in Canada by
J. B. Lippincott Company of
Canada Ltd, Toronto

Printed in Great Britain by
Billing & Sons Limited,
Guildford and London,
and bound by
Kemp Hall Bindery
Oxford

Contents

Preface

Spinal angiomas are relatively uncommon, and most practising neurologists and neurosurgeons have accumulated little personal experience of patients with such malformations. Until a few years ago, the treatment of these patients was usually futile, but recent refinements in neuroradiology have encouraged a more active and rational surgical approach to their management. In particular, the introduction of selective spinal angiography has permitted the accurate pre-operative delineation of these malformations, and this has allowed the aims of surgical treatment to be defined with greater precision. Perhaps as a consequence, recent reports from several neurological centres indicate that gratifying improvement may follow corrective surgery.

These developments indicate a change in the traditionally conservative management of patients with a spinal angioma. They emphasise the need for early recognition of these patients and for re-appraisal of the indications for their surgical treatment. Although an extensive literature is accumulating, it is disseminated among numerous medical journals and as such is not easily accessible to many practitioners. Moreover, most of these publications are concerned with small series of patients and deal with only a restricted aspect of the subject. Accordingly, my aim in writing this book has been to present a comprehensive account of spinal angiomas which, I hope, will be of value to those whose responsibility includes the care of such patients.

I would like to express my indebtedness to Dr P.C. Gautier-Smith for reading the manuscript and for his helpful advice, to Miss B.Laatz for her patient secretarial assistance, and to Miss P.Kingsland for her encouragement. I am grateful to Dr R.O.Barnard for his help with the section dealing with pathology and for providing illustrations; to Dr T.Powell for helpful discussion of the biophysical aspects of the subject; to Dr J.P.Patten for making the drawings; and to Mr Prentice and the Department of Medical Illustration at the Institute of Neurology, and Mr G.Cox and Mr T.Scott at Maida Vale Hospital for photographic assistance. I am particularly grateful to Professor Valentine Logue and Dr B.E.Kendall, each of whom contributed a chapter to this book and permitted me to include data from our jointly published work on some aspects of the subject. Such data were obtained by analysis of the case records of 60 patients with spinal angiomas, the great majority of whom were investigated at the National Hospitals for Nervous Diseases over the last 25 years. I am grateful to the consultant staff at these hospitals for permission to study their medical records, and to the Medical Committee of the National Hospitals for permission to publish this book.

Chapter 1
Introduction: the nature of spinal angiomas

The different forms of intradural spinal vascular hamartoma and tumour have, in the past, been designated by a bewildering variety of names. They have been categorised in turn on the basis of their macroscopic appearance, topographical relationships, microscopic structure, aetiology and pathological nature; in some cases, these individual parameters were combined to form further systems of classification which, by their very complexity, became a source of confusion. When viewed in their historical perspective, it is clear that these different classifications reflect the continuous evolution of thought on the subject. Nevertheless, the confusing nomenclature that resulted has become a hindrance, rather than an aid, to further progress.

Any general discussion of the various spinal vascular abnormalities is beyond the scope of the present work, but brief comment is necessary to clarify the nature of the anomaly under consideration. Cushing and Bailey (1928), in an analysis of cerebral lesions, recognised two broad groups comprising the vascular neoplasms (haemangioblastomas) and the vascular malformations (hamartomas). Their differentiation depended upon the presence in the latter of neural parenchyma as the interstitial component of the lesion, but Bergstrand (1936) correctly indicated that this did not necessarily apply in all cases. Nevertheless, such a division into two broad groups is of paramount importance and has received wide acceptance, Bergstrand's objection to it being met by the inclusion of cavernous angiomas—which have no neural interstitial tissue—as a separate subgroup of the hamartomas.

Histological examination of the hamartomas reveals no clear evidence of cellular proliferation, in contrast to the haemangioblastomas. Several types of hamartoma are recognised. The telangiectasis is a hamartoma in which local capillaries are pathologically enlarged. The cavernous angioma is considered by some (e.g. Michael and Levin, 1936) but not other authors (e.g. Russell and Rubinstein, 1959) to be a form of telangiectasis; it is usually a well-defined, purple, lobulated mass containing a tangled web of vascular spaces. These two forms of hamartoma are uncommon, particularly in relation to the spinal cord where they are usually of little clinical importance. Similarly, primary arterial aneurysms are exceedingly rare in vessels of the spinal cord and some authors doubt that they ever occur (Djindjian, Hurth and Houdart, 1970). These malformations will receive no further consideration here.

This book is concerned with the most common type of vascular hamartoma occurring in the spinal cord or within its leptomeninges, and this is customarily—but imprecisely—called a spinal angioma. Picturesquely likened to haemorrhoids by Gaupp (1888), it has also been referred to by a variety of other names including aneurysmal varix, cirsoid aneurysm, racemose venous angioma, and spinal or pial varicose veins. Spinal angiomas have been subdivided by several authors on the basis of their operative appearance or the pathological findings at autopsy, but Wyburn-Mason (1943) recognised only two main types. The *venous* type was said to consist of an abnormal mass of sinuous, turgid, blue pial veins localised mainly posteriorly below the mid-thoracic region of the cord. Microscopic examination revealed thick-walled pial vessels of abnormal structure, and marked proliferation of intramedullary capillaries, pre-capillaries and venules. The *arteriovenous* form consisted of a fistulous arteriovenous communication which bypassed the normal capillary bed, and was preferentially localised to either the region of the cervical enlargement anteriorly, or the lower part of the cord posteriorly. Inspection revealed large, tortuous arteries, in addition to distended veins, at one or other of these sites, and microscopic examination showed the presence of numerous vessels of different size and structure, some of which resembled arteries and veins. Wyburn-Mason also referred to a rarer primary arterial anomaly in which tortuous vessels, apparently arterial in nature, were present over the surface of the cord while draining veins were relatively inconspicuous, but other authors have usually classified this with the arteriovenous variety.

However, such a subdivision implies that these varieties are different in nature, whereas recent studies fail to support this concept. Thus, angiography has revealed only one type of abnormality in large series of patients, irrespective of the gross appearance of malformations at subsequent operation, and this consists essentially of an abnormal communication between the arterial and venous systems, without intervening capillaries (Houdart, Djindjian and Hurth, 1966; Di Chiro, Doppman and Ommaya, 1967; Baker, Love and Layton, 1967; Djindjian, Hurth and Houdart, 1970). Accordingly, although the fistulous nature of spinal angiomas may be more readily apparent at operation in some cases than in others, this presumably depends upon the volume of the shunt and the topographical relationship of the exposed vessels to the site of the abnormal arteriovenous communication rather than on any fundamental difference in the nature of the underlying malformation. Similarly, their subdivision on the basis of the pathological findings in excised specimens or at autopsy may be misleading because the vessels involved are often so deformed that arteries and veins cannot properly be distinguished, and in many cases only a small part of the malformation, which may not include the fistulous portion, is examined. Moreover, it may be impossible to recognise the site of the abnormal communication between arterial and venous systems unless a dye is injected into one of the involved arteries, and such a procedure is rarely undertaken.

Since venous and arteriovenous angiomas cannot be distinguished satisfactorily either angiographically or pathologically, they will be grouped together in this book under the unqualified term 'spinal angioma'. This may be reconciled with Wyburn-Mason's previous subdivision by suggesting that malformations with a shunt of large volume usually correspond to his so-called arteriovenous angiomas, while those with a shunt of small volume—in which it may be anticipated that the arterial components are morphologically less conspicuous—correspond to his venous variety. Circumstantial support for this view can be marshalled.

Wyburn-Mason (1943) found that in patients with arteriovenous malformations, initial symptoms often occur early in life, in contrast to patients with the venous type of angioma; moreover, in the former the malformation is frequently localised to the cervical region. At angiography, in contrast to angiomas in the thoracolumbar region, cervical malformations are usually found to have multiple arterial afferents (Houdart and Djindjian, 1966), suggesting a shunt of larger volume. Again, the angiographic appearance of a spinal vascular malformation is often strikingly different in young adults compared with older patients, irrespective of its location; multiple large feeding arteries are present and flow through the lesion is rapid, while in older age groups feeding vessels are less numerous and flow is usually slow (Ommaya, Di Chiro and Doppman, 1969). The implications of these differences will be considered further in later chapters.

By definition, spinal angiomas represent a presumed developmental anomaly and as such are congenital in nature, but this has not always been recognised. Kadyi (1889) related the morphological abnormalities to underlying infection, an aetiological factor which was subsequently incriminated in the development of subacute necrotic myelitis—a clinicopathological complication of spinal angiomas—by Foix and Alajouanine (1926). Clinical data to support such concepts were always lacking and recent observations, discussed above, now make them untenable. The possib!e role of trauma in the development of these vascular anomalies is more difficult to define. It is certainly true that in a few patients symptoms have developed soon, sometimes almost immediately, after trauma (Sargent, 1925; Aminoff and Logue, 1974a), but this does not indicate that trauma led to the development of the fistula; it may merely have modified flow through a pre-existing shunt by influencing regional blood flow. Moreover, it may well be that symptoms were due in some cases to the trauma itself, and not to the angioma which was discovered incidentally during the course of neuro-radiological investigation.

Other congenital anomalies have sometimes been described in patients with a spinal angioma. The significance of such associations will be considered further in Chapter 3.

Chapter 2
The spinal circulation

Spinal angiomas represent a developmental anomaly of the spinal circulatory system. Accordingly, the proper study of these malformations requires an appreciation of the normal development and anatomy of the vascular supply to the spinal cord. Since much that has been written on this subject is either incomplete or inaccurate, a detailed account is given here.

Development

EXTRAMEDULLARY ARTERIES

When blood vessels begin to extend beyond their primary location in the walls of the yolk sac and gut, the first foetal structure that they vascularise is the neural tube. The dorsal intersegmental arteries develop as offshoots from the aorta, and extend along the spinal roots to reach the neural tube; each then divides into dorsal and ventral branches, which form a lateral vascular plexus in the 5-week-old foetus. Anastomoses occur between vessels in adjacent segments, forming an irregular, longitudinally-orientated plexus within which a single channel, the primitive arterial tract, develops ventrally on each side. In time, these paired tracts are converted into a single anterior spinal artery by their medial displacement and eventual fusion (Torr, 1957). Paired, longitudinal, posterior spinal arteries similarly develop in the lateral vascular plexuses, in close proximity to the posterior nerve roots; other inconstant, and frequently incomplete, longitudinal arterial tracts may also develop posteriorly. Concomitant with the development of the anterior and posterior spinal arteries, vessels in the lateral plexuses differentiate into arteries which join the main longitudinal channels at each segmental level, both anteriorly and posteriorly. There are thus 31 paired segmental arteries in the early foetus, their number decreasing during the further development of the embryo.

The primary distribution of the dorsal intersegmental arteries to the spinal cord is soon altered by the development of an additional branch to supply the somites and body wall. This anterior branch enlarges to such an extent that the original posterior vessel to the cord eventually appears merely as a minor offshoot (Arey, 1965).

The paired serial symmetry of the early embryo now becomes profoundly altered due to fusion, obliteration and differential enlargement of vessels, and to the development of new vessels and pathways. A number of longitudinal anastomoses form between the intersegmental arteries. A pre-costal anastomosis develops in front of the head and neck of each rib (or the costal element of the vertebrae), a post-costal anastomosis forms dorsal to the neck of each rib, and a post-transverse anastomosis comes to lie behind the transverse processes. The trunks of origin of each of the upper six cervical intersegmental arteries atrophy, and the post-costal anastomosis between these vessels enlarges to form that portion of the vertebral artery that runs within the foramina transversariae; this artery thus appears to originate from the stem of the 7th cervical intersegmental artery. In parenthesis, it may be noted that there is some discord in the literature on this point, due to differences in terminology. Some authors follow Padget (1954) in not numbering among the cervical series the dorsal intersegmental artery which accompanies the 1st cervical nerve, because it does not pass between two cervical segments. Using this nomenclature, the vertebral artery will appear to arise from the stem of the 6th cervical intersegmental artery, and will comprise the post-costal anastomoses of this vessel with the upper 5 cervical, and the suboccipital, intersegmental arteries.

In the cervical and upper thoracic regions, the pre-costal anastomosis forms the thyrocervical trunk and the superior intercostal stem, while the post-transverse anastomosis develops into the deep cervical artery. In the rest of the thoracic region, and in the upper lumbar region, the intersegmental arteries remain as serially-arranged intercostal and lumbar vessels originating from the aorta. In the lumbo-sacral region, the umbilical artery on each side forms anastomotic connections with the 5th lumbar intersegmental artery, and its original connection with the dorsal aorta then atrophies until it appears to arise from the intersegmental stem. The external and internal iliac arteries arise as branches of this stem. Anastomotic communications of the sacral intersegmental arteries with the internal iliac artery on each side increase in importance until these intersegmental arteries appear to originate from it; the dorsal aorta accordingly becomes much smaller in this region, forming the middle sacral artery which terminates in the glomus coccygeum, a curious arteriovenous anastomosis (Hamilton and Mossman, 1972).

INTRAMEDULLARY ARTERIES

The first vessels to penetrate the developing cord are sprouts extending dorsally from the primitive tracts.

On reaching the level of the roof of the central canal, they divide into anterior and posterior branches. As the paired primitive arterial tracts become converted into the single anterior spinal artery, the sprouts become transformed into the central arteries of the cord. Anastomoses are established between branches of these arteries and vessels which grow in from the dorsal and lateral surfaces of the cord, to form a plexus around the ependyma. By about the 4th month of gestation, capillaries are distributed equally throughout the grey and the white matter, but in the following months there is a relative increase in the vascularity of the former.

VEINS

The veins also develop in the lateral vascular plexus on each side, and segmental vessels draining through the intervertebral foramina are soon established anteriorly. This is followed by the development of paired, longitudinal, antero-median veins, which accompany the anterior spinal artery and drain laterally into the segmental veins. The posterior part of the vascular plexus drains by segmental vessels, which run with the posterior nerve roots and drain also the longitudinal posterior spinal veins which form just posterior to these roots.

Adult configuration

EXTRAMEDULLARY ARTERIES

The foetal, segmental supply to the longitudinal, anterior and posterior spinal arteries is modified during the later development of the embryo so that, well before 6 months gestation, only a limited number of so-called lateral spinal arteries—which pass through the intervertebral foramina with the nerve roots—continue to supply the spinal cord. These lateral spinal arteries give off branches to the paravertebral muscles, dura and vertebrae, in addition to 'radicular' arteries of three types, as shown in Figure 2.1. The radicular arteries (anterior and posterior) *sensu strictiori* supply the nerve roots, and the radiculo-pial arteries extend to the pial-leptomeningeal arterial plexus; both may be regarded as vestiges of arteries which originally contributed to the spinal cord circulation. The anterior and posterior radiculo-medullary, or medullary, arteries are the only vessels which continue to make a meaningful contribution to the blood supply of the cord, and they only occur at certain

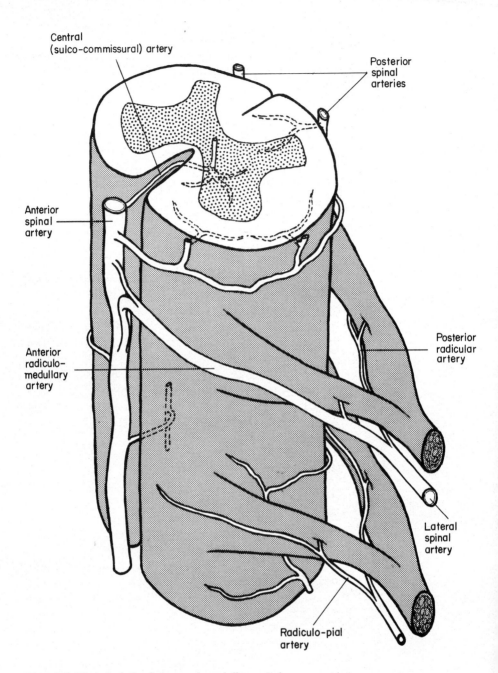

Figure 2.1. The spinal circulation: extramedullary arteries.
The lateral spinal arteries which traverse the intervertebral
foramina give off radicular arteries to the nerve roots,
radiculo-pial arteries to the leptomeningeal arterial plexus,
and radiculo-medullary arteries which supply the cord via
the anterior and posterior spinal arteries.

segmental levels, which vary in different individuals. Anterior and posterior radiculo-medullary arteries may contribute to their respective longitudinal spinal arteries at the same segmental level, but this is not usual (Gillilan, 1958).

The radiculo-medullary arteries which join the anterior spinal artery usually number between 6 and 10 (Kadyi, 1889; Suh and Alexander, 1939; Gillilan, 1958), 0–6 supplying the cervical region, 2–4 the thoracic region and 1 or 2 the lumbar area. Some authors cite higher figures, due to a failure to appreciate that many 'radicular' arteries do not reach the cord. The anterior radiculo-medullary arteries vary in diameter between 0·2 and 0·8 mm, but the great anterior artery to the lumbar enlargement is appreciably larger (1·0–1·3 mm). Radiculo-medullary arteries joining with the posterior spinal vessels number between 10 and 23, and vary in diameter between 0·2 and 0·5 mm.

The anterior spinal artery lies within the pia and extends the length of the cord, supplying its anterior two-thirds. It may be duplicated for short distances in the cervical region due to incomplete fusion of its two foetal precursors. The radiculo-medullary vessels joining it bifurcate to give a branch passing upward and another bending sharply downward. It may thus be considered to comprise the terminal branches of successive anterior radiculo-medullary arteries (Turnbull, 1972). At any given level, it is narrowest at a point mid-way between the nearest rostral and caudal feeding vessels (Suh and Alexander, 1939). The main branches from it are the radial and central arteries.

The posterior spinal arteries are paired, longitudinal, plexiform vessels, variable in size, running in relation to the posterior nerve roots. Originating from the intra-cranial portion of the vertebral artery or from the posterior inferior cerebellar artery on each side, they supply the posterior one-third of the cord, as they descend its length.

The anterior spinal artery varies markedly in calibre along its length, being narrowest in the upper thoracic region and again just rostral to its junction with the great anterior radiculo-medullary artery, where it is sometimes discontinuous. Similarly, the posterior spinal arteries are not always the continuous vessels classically described, but are irregular, incomplete chains (Suh and Alexander, 1939), which are occasionally interrupted in the thoracic region. These observations, and the results of more recent studies performed in his laboratories, led Lazorthes and his colleagues (1958) to conclude that there are three main arterial territories in the vertical axis of the spinal cord, with little functional anastomosis between them. These territories, which are indicated in Figure 2.2, merit individual consideration.

(a) *The cervico-thoracic region*, which is richly vascularised, comprises the cervical and first 2 or 3 thoracic segments of the cord. Its radiculo-medullary arteries arise from branches of the subclavian arteries, but their precise origin is variable. The vertebral arteries, during their intracranial course, give off paired anterior spinal rami which fuse to form the rostral part of the anterior spinal artery. Lazorthes (1972) believes that this part rarely descends below the 4th cervical segment, but this does not accord with the findings in other recent studies (Bolton, 1939; Adams and van Geertruyden, 1956). The anterior spinal circulation also receives 2 or 3 radiculo-medullary branches from the vertebrals as they ascend in the foramina transversariae, the most constant of these passing through the 3rd cervical intervertebral foramen. Another vessel, which joins it relatively constantly, arises from one of the branches of the costocervical trunks (superior intercostal and deep cervical arteries) and enters usually through the 6th or 7th intervertebral foramen. Branches from the occipital, deep cervical and ascending cervical arteries form a suboccipital anastomotic plexus with branches of the vertebral arteries, and may contribute to the arterial supply of this portion of the cord (Lazorthes, Gouazé, Bastide, Santini, Zadeh and Burdin, 1966). The posterior spinal arteries are often fed by a radiculo-medullary vessel in each segment of the cervical enlargement, but there may be no feeding vessels from the 8th cervical to the 4th thoracic segments (Tureen, 1938).

(b) *The mid-thoracic region*, comprising the 4th to 8th thoracic segments, is supplied by branches from the serially-arranged intercostal arteries. Its anterior spinal circulation is usually fed by only a single radiculo-medullary artery while its posterior circulation may be supplied by 2 or 3 segmental vessels.

(c) *The thoraco-lumbar region* comprises the remainder of the cord, including the lumbar enlargement. It is fed by radiculo-medullary branches from the intercostal and lumbar arteries. The main supply to the anterior circulation is from the great anterior radiculo-medullary artery (Adamkiewicz, 1882) which enters most frequently from the left side. It accompanies the 10th, 11th or 12th thoracic roots in 75 per cent of individuals, one of the

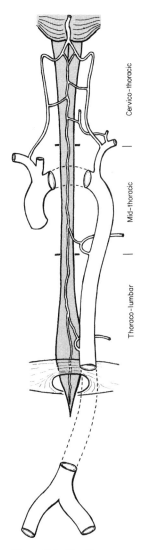

Cervico-thoracic

Mid-thoracic

Thoraco-lumbar

Figure 2.2. The three arterial territories in the vertical axis of the spinal cord, showing the main arterial supply to the anterior spinal artery in each region. Full details are given in the text.

3 more rostral roots in 15 per cent, and either the 1st or 2nd lumbar root in the remaining 10 per cent; it passes upward with the nerve root, continuing on to reach the anterior median fissure where it turns caudally at an acute angle. When its origin is high, another vessel—the artery of the conus medullaris—supplies the anterior spinal artery at a lower level (Lazorthes, Gouazé, Bastide, Soutoul, Zadeh and Santini, 1966). There are usually several posterior radiculo-medullary arteries to this region, one of which may originate from the same stem as the great anterior vessel. At the conus the anterior and posterior spinal arteries are linked by the cruciate anastomosis, to which small arteries supplying the sacral roots may contribute. These vessels arise from the iliolumbar and lateral sacral arteries (which are branches of the internal iliac), and the lumbar and middle sacral arteries. This anastomosis may be of importance in the event of obstruction to the main radiculo-medullary vessel supplying the anterior spinal artery in the thoraco-lumbar region.

At all levels arterial branches which supply the paraspinal muscles or vertebral bodies anastomose with corresponding branches from adjacent segments to form a paravertebral plexus extending from the occiput to the sacrum (Lazorthes and Gouazé, 1968; Lazorthes, 1972).

INTRAMEDULLARY ARTERIES

The anatomical arrangement of the intramedullary arteries is shown in Figure 2.3, and the distribution of blood within the spinal cord is indicated in Figure 2.4. It can be seen that branches of the anterior and posterior spinal arteries form a fine plexus around the cord. From this plexus and its parent vessels, radially-orientated branches are given off, and blood flows centripetally through these to supply much of the white matter and the posterior horns of grey matter. The largest branches of the anterior spinal artery are, however, the central or sulco-commissural arteries which arise in the anterior median fissure and penetrate the cord; blood passes through these vessels to the grey matter (except the posterior horns) and the innermost portion of the white. The central arteries are larger and more numerous in the cervical and lumbar cord than in the thoracic, and branches from each overlap with those from the adjacent vessels. They do not usually bifurcate, but turn to one or other side of the cord (Tureen, 1938; Herren and Alexander, 1939).

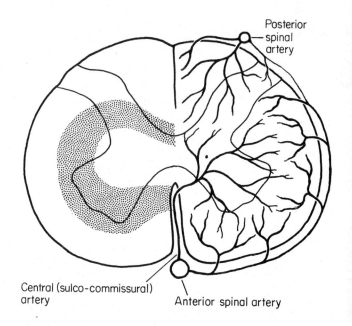

Figure 2.3. Transverse section of the cord showing the intramedullary arterial circulation. The anatomical arrangement of the intramedullary arteries is shown on the right of the figure. Radially orientated branches from the pial plexus around the cord supply much of the white matter, and the posterior horns of grey matter. The central or sulco-commissural arteries arise from the anterior spinal artery, and supply the grey matter (except the posterior horns) and the innermost portion of the white. The stippled region shown on the left represents the area of cord which is supplied from both sources.

Posterior spinal artery

Central (sulco-commissural) artery

Anterior spinal artery

In general, the grey matter is more richly vascularised than the white, but its vascularity shows marked regional variation. Thus, Craigie (1972) cites unpublished studies in the cat by Brightman demonstrating that the vascularity of grey matter is greatest in the lumbar region and least in the thoracic. Fazio (1939) observed that capillary networks increased in density in areas of grey matter containing high cell counts. The capillary plexus is continuous within the cord, but during life this anastomosis is inadequate to function as an effective collateral system of physiological importance (Gillilan, 1958).

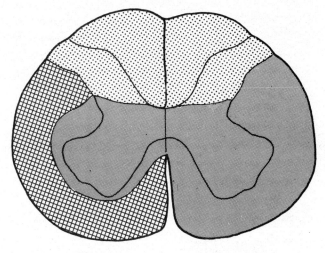

Figure 2.4. Transverse section of the cord, showing its blood supply. The lightly-stippled region is supplied by the posterior spinal arteries, and the darkly-stippled region by the anterior spinal artery. The cross-hatched area to the left of the figure indicates the region fed by radial branches supplied from the anterior spinal circulation.

The anatomy of the venous system draining the cord had largely been neglected until the detailed study of Gillilan (1970), on which the present account is based. An antero-median group of intrinsic veins drains the capillaries of the grey and white commissures, medial cell columns of the anterior horns, and white matter of the anterior funiculi; it empties through the central veins into the anterior median spinal vein, which runs longitudinally in the anterior median fissure. The remainder of the cord drains through radial veins to the coronal (pial) vessels, the most prominent of which run longitudinally over the posterior and lateral surfaces of the cord. Figure 2.5 shows the arrangement and drainage of the intramedullary veins.

The anterior median spinal vein drains the central veins and the small anterior and antero-lateral coronal veins running in the pia. It may be duplicated in part, especially in the cervical or thoracic regions. The posterior coronal veins, often huge, usually form a convoluted plexus that becomes increasingly tortuous with advancing age; their pattern is variable, but some tend to run over the posterior median and intermediate sulci, or along the line of entrance of the posterior nerve roots. The coronal plexus lying laterally between the anterior and posterior nerve roots is of particular interest in that there are few anastomotic connections between its anterior and posterior halves in the upper two-thirds of the cord.

The superficial veins around the cord drain in turn by the medullary veins which accompany the nerve roots (Figure 2.5). There are between 8 and 14 anteriorly, and more posteriorly, especially in the cervical region; higher figures have been given by earlier authors, who probably failed to differentiate between veins draining the cord and those draining only a nerve root. The anterior medullary veins drain the anterior median spinal vein and the coronal veins in the anterior half of the cord, while the posterior medullary veins drain the posterior and postero-lateral coronal vessels. The medullary veins show no correlation, in their size and location, with the medullary arteries. However, among the roots of the cauda equina it is usually possible to recognise a relatively large vein descending on the left side from one of the segments between the 11th thoracic and 3rd lumbar; this is generally referred to as the great anterior medullary vein.

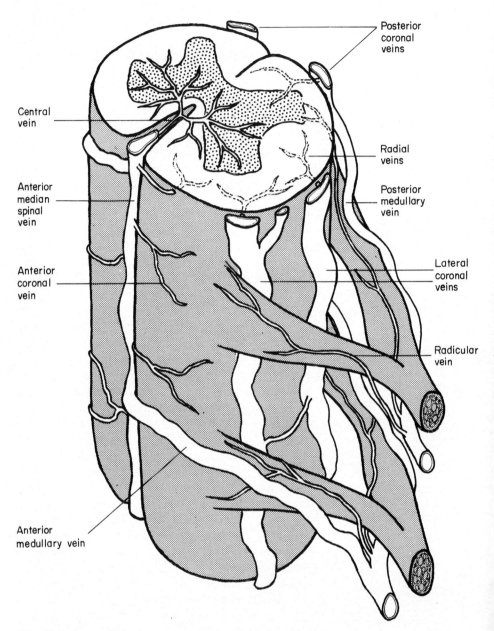

Central
vein

Anterior
median
spinal
vein

Anterior
coronal
vein

Anterior
medullary vein

Posterior
coronal
veins

Radial
veins

Posterior
medullary
vein

Lateral
coronal
veins

Radicular
vein

Figure 2.5. Venous drainage of the spinal cord. The antero-medial part of the cord drains through the central veins to the anterior median spinal vein, while the remainder drains through radial veins to the coronal (pial) vessels, the most prominent of which run longitudinally over the posterior and lateral surfaces of the cord.

The anterior and posterior medullary veins pass to the intervertebral foramina, where radicular veins draining the nerve roots, and segmental communications from the anterior and posterior epidural and paravertebral plexuses, also converge. The direction of blood flow in the medullary veins is outward to the intervertebral veins, which pass through the intervertebral foramina and drain the interconnected epidural and paravertebral plexuses. These veins end, in turn, in the vertebral, posterior intercostal, lumbar and lateral sacral veins. In addition, the longitudinal spinal veins and the epidural venous plexus communicate rostrally with intracranial veins and dural sinuses.

Application

No apology is made for providing such a detailed account of the spinal circulatory system, since many clinicians are unfamiliar with recent studies on the subject and a few may still entertain the classical, but inaccurate, notion of three continuous, longitudinal spinal arteries supplied by radiculo-medullary vessels of equal importance. Moreover, several aspects of the normal development and anatomy of the spinal vasculature are directly relevant to any study of spinal angiomas.

In the course of development, segmental arteries and veins develop from the lateral capillary plexus on each side. Initially they are not structurally distinct, but are named in anticipation of the particular vessels they are destined to form. The factors determining this differentiation of vessels and the direction of normal pathways are not fully known, but mechanical and haemodynamic factors are probably important. Whether spinal angiomas develop at this early stage through the formation of unusual pathways in the primitive lateral vascular plexus, or later due to incomplete development of vessels, disappearance of vessels normally retained, fusion and absorption of vessels, or by some other means, is uncertain. It must, however, be noted that spinal angiomas occur more commonly in the thoraco-lumbar region than elsewhere, and are usually situated posteriorly. The posterior spinal circulation is normally established a little later than the anterior, and the circulation to the cord similarly develops later in caudal regions than in more rostral areas. The preferential location of spinal angiomas may, therefore, relate to the time of their development.

Of more immediate importance is the observation that of the 62 segmental arteries contributing to the intra-medullary circulation of the early foetus, over half subsequently regress, providing a blood supply only to the nerve roots or pia. If an angioma is supplied by abnormal vessels of this type, the circulation through it may well remain distinct from that to the cord itself, thereby permitting its surgical treatment.

Recent angiographic and operative findings (Kaufman, Ommaya, Di Chiro and Doppman, 1970; Shephard, 1965;

Logue, Aminoff and Kendall, 1974), confirm that most spinal angiomas are supplied by one or more of the radiculo-pial arteries, and only a minority are supplied either partly or completely by radiculo-medullary vessels. Their feeding vessels usually accompany the posterior nerve roots, but may sometimes arise anteriorly, particularly in the cervical region. Their venous drainage, either directly or indirectly, is to the longitudinally orientated coronal veins, which are often markedly distended and tortuous when viewed at operation or post-mortem.

The pre-operative delineation of these malformations has been guided by the detailed descriptions of the spinal circulatory system provided by anatomists, and by an appreciation of the multiplicity and variability of the normal arterial supply to the cord. Neuro-radiological investigation is directed to visualising the angioma and to defining its situation, feeding vessels, and the local arterial supply to the cord itself. This may necessitate extensive angiographic studies if the malformation is situated in the cervical region, because of the numerous feeding and anastomotic vessels normally found in this area, or if it is located in the lumbar region, because ascending vessels from the lumbar and lateral sacral arteries may contribute to the circulation there. The diverse sources of the normal blood supply to these two regions can only be understood by reference to the manner of their embryological development. In the thoraco-lumbar region, the intramedullary circulation depends predominantly on a single source, the great anterior radiculo-medullary artery of Adamkiewicz, which must always be visualised. The feasibility of surgically correcting a spinal angioma, and the manner in which this may be attained most satisfactorily, will depend on the information derived from angiography.

There is some difference of opinion as to the mechanism responsible for the steadily progressive and extensive neurological involvement which occurs in many patients with these malformations. This will be discussed in some detail in a later chapter, but it may be noted here that recent studies relate it to the pattern of the intramedullary venous drainage (Gillilan, 1970; Aminoff, Barnard and Logue, 1974).

One final point must be made. In patients with coarctation of the aorta there is enlargement of the collateral vessels connecting parts of the aorta above and below the narrowed segment. This may involve the spinal circulation; blood enters the anterior spinal artery rostrally, and then descends to pass back to the aorta through radiculo-medullary branches below the level of the coarctation. In these circumstances, patients may develop signs of spinal cord dysfunction (Wyburn-Mason, 1943); at myelography or operation, the distended, tortuous, collateral vessels may mistakenly be attributed to a spinal vascular malformation, in spite of their obvious arterial character, unless the coarctation is recognised or angiography is performed.

Chapter 3
Associated lesions

In the preceding chapters spinal angiomas were related to the maldevelopment of one or more of the segmental arteries which originally supplied the spinal cord. It is not altogether surprising, therefore, that they may be associated with other developmental vascular anomalies.

Cutaneous angiomas

The most common association recorded in the literature is with cutaneous angiomas, and these are often said to be situated within the same metameric segment as the spinal lesion. Some of the earlier reported cases are difficult to assess because of the confusion in terminology referred to in Chapter 1, and it is frequently impossible, from the descriptions provided, to relate them to modern classifications. The case reported by Berenbruch (1890)—the first in which spinal and cutaneous lesions were segmentally related—exemplifies this problem. The patient, a 16-year-old boy with a spastic paraplegia, was found to have three superficial angiolipomas, two of which were connected by a plexus of veins with an epidural angioma, and an intramedullary vascular lesion whose nature is not entirely clear; later authors have referred to 'cord tumor' (Cobb, 1915), 'intra-medullary telangiectasis' (Wyburn-Mason, 1943), and 'venous angioma' (Kissel and Dureux, 1972) in discussing this case. Accordingly, cases such as this have been excluded from the present discussion, as have those in which the nature of the spinal lesion was not confirmed by radiological, operative or post-mortem study.

The earliest satisfactorily documented case in which a spinal angioma was associated with a cutaneous angioma involving the same metameric segment is probably that of Cobb (1915). This case is of particular interest for historical reasons and because a correct pre-operative neurological diagnosis was made (by Dr Harvey Cushing) on the basis of the cutaneous lesion. In brief, the patient, an 8-year-old boy, developed sudden, severe back pain, weakness and numbness in the legs, incontinence of faeces and retention of urine. He was admitted to hospital and subsequently seen by Dr Cushing, whose notes, cited by Cobb (1915), read:

'This child shows a transverse paraplegia with the upper level of anaesthesia about at the tenth thoracic level. It has been presumed, owing to the acute onset of symptoms, that the case was one of poliomyelitis of unusual type. However, the definite upper level of anaes-thesia, the complete lower limb paralysis with exaggerated reflexes, visceral paralysis, and priapism, make it fairly definite that there must be pressure against the cord. Examination shows a slight scoliosis with prominence of the spinal muscles at the scapula level, and over the lower portion of the right scapula there is a naevus about 5 inches in diameter. The presumptive diagnosis is of a congenital lesion pressing upon the cord, either a dermoid or an angioma. Similar meningeal angiomata have been observed by myself in association with facial naevi.'

Cushing's operative note, which provides a useful description of the lesion, is also quoted by Cobb, and reads in part as follows:

'A long median incision was made with removal of the laminae, possibly from T6 to T10 inclusive. . . . The exposed dura was tense, bulging, and transmitted an unusually dark subdural coloration. Fortunately great pains were taken to enter the dura without injuring the arachnoid, for a careless entrance would certainly have injured some of the enormous vessels which were disclosed on opening the meninx. Such of the arachnoid membrane as could be identified was more or less adherent to the dura by fine adhesions which readily broke down as the dura was drawn to each side. This exposed an extraordinary tangle of huge pulsating vessels filling the canal. . . . It seemed futile to attempt to ligate any of the vessels. . . .'

Since this early report there have been occasional accounts of other patients with coexistent cutaneous angiomas involving, in part at least, the same metameric segments as the spinal lesion, and situated usually over the trunk (Sterling and Jakimowicz, 1936; Turner and Kernohan, 1941; Wyburn-Mason, 1943; Cross, 1947; Trupp and Sachs, 1948; van Bogaert, 1950; Gilbert, 1952; Henson and Croft, 1956; Nielsen, Marvin and Seletz, 1958; Fine, 1961; Strain, 1964; Szojchet, 1968; Doppman, Wirth, Di Chiro and Ommaya, 1969; Djindjian, Hurth and Houdart, 1970). The number of patients with such coexistent lesions is small, and Aminoff and Logue (1974a) found no record of this association in any of the 60 patients with a spinal angioma whose case notes they studied. Although less than 30 instances of this association have, in fact, been satisfactorily documented in the literature, many of these were derived from two recently published series in which it occurred in 21 per cent (Doppman, Wirth, Di Chiro and Ommaya, 1969) and 12 per cent (Djindjian, Hurth and Houdart, 1970) of patients. Moreover, in 2 of the patients in the former series the cutaneous angioma, which was in the midline, was not readily apparent on casual inspection, but became conspicuous when the patients performed a Valsalva manoeuvre. This suggests that the more meticulous scrutiny of patients, combined with use of the Valsalva manoeuvre as an aid to the visualisation of inconspicuous cutaneous lesions, may enable this association to be recognised more frequently than hitherto.

DEVELOPMENTAL BASIS OF THIS ASSOCIATION

Cobb (1915), in agreement with earlier writers who emphasised the occurrence of angiomas in relation to territories of cutaneous innervation, concluded that they arise from a developmental fault of the central nervous system. Wyburn-Mason (1943) rejected this view, emphasising that extradural and vertebral lesions can similarly be associated with metameric cutaneous angiomas. He attributed the association of spinal and segmentally-related cutaneous angiomas to a developmental disorder of the 'whole neuro-myo-dermatome', the lesions being independent of each other. Neither of these views seems entirely satisfactory, however, and it is more likely that this association is related to the common segmental origin of their blood supply when the cutaneous lesion is situated on the trunk. In other words, there is an early disorder of the embryonic development of blood vessels arising at a particular segmental level.

During the course of foetal development the primitive segmental vessels to the cord become greatly modified; branches are developed to supply other structures, while many of the original arteries regress so that they subsequently fail to supply the intramedullary circulation. Nevertheless, the primitive serial symmetry of the intersegmental arteries persists throughout life in the thoracic and upper lumbar region, as indicated in Chapter 2. In contrast, the development of the vertebral and iliac arteries leads to considerable modification of the early segmental pattern in the cervical and lumbo-sacral regions. Moreover, branches from the 7th cervical and 5th lumbar intersegmental arteries enlarge to form the axial vessels of the upper and lower limbs. Nerves at the level of each limb-bud grow into its mesenchyme, becoming distributed to the differentiating muscles and to the skin in a segmental manner. In spite of their innervation, the limb muscles are not derived from segmental somites, but develop *in situ*; similarly, much of the dermis differentiates from non-specific mesenchyme subjacent to the epidermis

20   *Chapter 3*

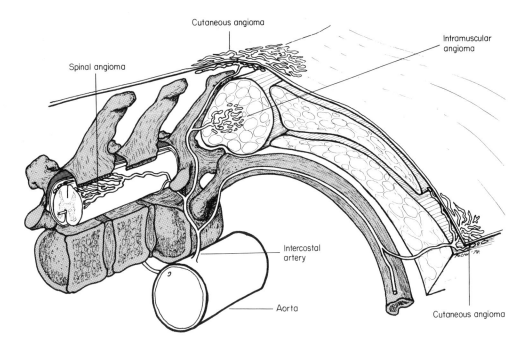

Cutaneous angioma

Spinal angioma

Intramuscular angioma

Intercostal artery

Aorta

Cutaneous angioma

Figure 3.1. Spinal, cutaneous and intramuscular angiomas, supplied from the same segmental source. As illustrated in this case, cutaneous and intramuscular angiomas do not necessarily overlie the spinal lesion.

(Murray, 1928; Arey, 1965). Accordingly, maldevelopment of 'the whole neuro-myo-dermatome' cannot explain the association of a spinal angioma with a similar cutaneous lesion over the limbs, since the limbs do not have a segmental origin.

In many of the earlier reports detailing this association, selective spinal angiography was not performed, and neither the origin of vessels feeding the spinal lesion nor the segmental level of the shunt itself can be established with certainty. Analysis of these cases reveals that in most instances the cutaneous angioma was situated over the posterior surface of the trunk, within the territory supplied by the segmental arterial stem from which the feeding vessel to the spinal lesion probably originated. More recently, visualisation of a spinal vascular malformation and an associated cutaneous angioma was achieved in 6 patients by selective catheterisation of the same intercostal or lumbar artery (Doppman, Wirth, Di Chiro and Ommaya, 1969), confirming the common segmental origin of the blood supply to both lesions, as shown in Figure 3.1.

CUTANEOUS ANGIOMAS OVER THE LIMBS

In patients with a spinal angioma, any coexistent cutaneous vascular malformation is usually situated over the trunk, at least in part, but it may sometimes involve the limbs. Thus, in 3 cases (Wyburn-Mason, 1943; Henson and Croft, 1956; Fine, 1961) an extensive cutaneous vascular lesion involving one or both arms was associated with a cervical spinal angioma. In the case described by Henson and Croft (1956) a vascular malformation involving the first 4 cervical segments of the cord was associated with a cutaneous angioma in the left upper limb and thorax. In the other 2 cases the cutaneous angioma was similarly very extensive, while the level of the spinal lesion was not defined by the angiographic location of the shunt or origin of its feeding vessels, but related merely to the topographical extent of abnormal vessels over the surface of the cord.

The diffuse distribution of one or both lesions in these cases makes it difficult to ascertain the extent to which they corresponded segmentally. Furthermore, in the patient reported by Fine (1961) there was an abnormal fistulous communication between the arteries and veins of the right forearm in addition to extensive cutaneous angiomas. Although the blood supply to the vascular lesions in these cases relates embryologically to the stem of the same (7th cervical) primitive intersegmental artery, this relationship is less obvious than in patients with a coexistent cutaneous angioma situated on the trunk. Moreover, it seems less likely that this relationship has any relevance to the association of such lesions, since many of the named arteries in the limbs are formed *in situ* comparatively late in development as new vessels which link up with the original axial vessel. One further case should, however, be mentioned. Gilbert (1952) reported a patient who had a cervical spinal angioma, a segmentally-related cutaneous one, and numerous small angiomas in the omentum. This is of particular interest since the coeliac trunk—which in part supplies the omentum—probably represents the original splanchnic segmental vessels of the 7th cervical segment (Hamilton and Mossman, 1972). Whether such correlations are of any significance is difficult to determine, however, and additional case reports must be awaited before further conclusions are drawn.

In at least 2 cases (Sterling and Jakimowicz, 1936; Wyburn-Mason, 1943) a discrete cutaneous angioma in the lower limbs has been found to coexist with a spinal vascular malformation which extended over the surface of several segments in the lower part of the cord, but was not defined angiographically. The data available are insufficient to allow further discussion of these cases.

There are several important implications of this association of spinal and cutaneous angiomas. In the first place, the presence of a cutaneous angioma over the trunk in a patient with a myelopathy and/or radiculopathy of uncertain aetiology may suggest the correct diagnosis, as in the case reported by Cobb (1915). Similarly, in a patient with subarachnoid haemorrhage, some of the clinical features may indicate a spinal source, the nature of which is suggested by a cutaneous vascular lesion over the trunk or limbs (Henson and Croft, 1956). Secondly, the presence of a cutaneous angioma on the trunk may aid the angiographic investigation of a patient suspected to have a spinal angioma, particularly when the neurological signs are unhelpful in localising the lesion. Thus, the location of the cutaneous lesion may suggest both the side and the level at which segmental vessels should be injected first to identify the arteries feeding the spinal angioma. Thirdly, the surgical management of the patient may be influenced by the presence of the cutaneous angioma, as in a striking example that was reported recently. A 16-year-old boy was found to have a mid-thoracic spinal angioma and a huge, overlying cutaneous angioma which precluded laminectomy; fortunately it was possible to obliterate the spinal lesion by percutaneous embolisation (Doppman, Di Chiro and Ommaya, 1968). It must not be assumed, however, that the cutaneous angioma will necessarily overlie the spinal lesion; the segmental arteries to the cord normally ascend a variable distance from their level of entry into the spinal canal, because of the disproportionate growth of the vertebral column in relation to the spinal cord during foetal development (Figure 3.1).

The significance of cutaneous angiomas must be interpreted with some caution. They may occur in a non-segmental distribution in some patients with a spinal angioma (Alexander, 1922; Wyburn-Mason, 1943; Doppman, Wirth, Di Chiro and Ommaya, 1969; Djindjian, Hurth and Houdart, 1970; Aminoff and Logue, 1974a), and may also be associated with other types of spinal vascular hamartoma, and with epidural and vertebral angiomas, in either a segmental or non-segmental manner.

Angiomas in the paraspinal muscles

As is shown in Figure 3.1, arteries to the paraspinal muscles originate from the same segmental stem as arteries entering the spinal canal. It is surprising, therefore, that the association of a spinal angioma with a similar lesion in the paraspinal muscles has seldom been recorded.

Turner and Kernohan (1941) reported a patient with spinal, cutaneous and intramuscular angiomas, all of which were apparently related segmentally although their precise location was not described. More recently, Pia (1973) has emphasised the occasional occurrence of vascular malformations involving all the contiguous layers between the subarachnoid space and subcutaneous tissues except for the dura itself.

This association may have important practical implications. Sargent (1925) was obliged to abandon an exploratory laminectomy in one of his patients because of haemorrhage from numerous dilated, tortuous, thin-walled arteries which permeated the overlying muscles and bone. The patient died shortly after the operation, and post-mortem examination confirmed the presence of a spinal angioma in the cervical region.

Epidural and vertebral angiomas

As might have been anticipated from the normal regional blood supply, a spinal angioma may be associated with an epidural (van Bogaert, 1950; Newquist and Mayfield, 1960; Pia, 1973) or vertebral angioma (Roger, Paillas, Bonnal and Vigoureux, 1951; Girard and Garde, 1955; Arseni and Samitca, 1959; Newman, 1959; Aminoff and Logue, 1974a). Although a vertebral angioma is usually recognised radiologically by the reticular appearance of the vertebral body, plain X-rays may be normal, the anomaly being recognised at angiography or by histological examination. By these means a vertebral angioma was recognised in 5 out of 56 patients with a spinal angioma who were studied angiographically, and in all cases it was located at the segmental level corresponding to the spinal lesion (Djindjian, Hurth and Houdart, 1970); in 2 cases, cutaneous, vertebral and spinal angiomas were coexistent.

More widespread vascular anomalies

In 2 patients an angiographically-defined spinal angioma is reported to have occurred in association with clinical manifestations of the Osler–Weber–Rendu syndrome, and in both cases other family members were known to have telangiectasia of the skin and mucous membranes (Djindjian, Hurth and Houdart, 1970).

Varicose leg veins developing at an unusually early age have been reported in a few patients. One of Wyburn-Mason's (1943) patients had suffered from varicose veins since the age of 12 years; his brother had developed similar varicosities when aged 8 years, and his father, grandfather and great grandfather had also been affected at a very early age. Similarly, a patient reported by Djindjian, Hurth and Houdart (1970) had developed varicose leg veins in early childhood; presenting with subarachnoid haemor hage at the age of 12 years, he was found to have three spinal angiomatous malformations, a vertebral angioma and an arteriovenous fistula in the region of the femoral vessels.

In several instances a visceral angioma has been reported in patients with a spinal angioma. However, whether this association occurs more frequently than by chance is uncertain, since angiomas are not uncommonly found in the viscera, particularly the liver.

Lymphatic anomalies

A patient with multiple congenital anomalies, including lymphatic dysplasia, has recently come to the author's attention through the kindness of Dr R.E.Kelly, and merits brief discussion. At the age of 12 years the patient was found to have a cutaneous angioma at the right ankle and diffuse, multiple, abnormal arteriovenous fistulae in the right leg and thigh. Two years later he had a series of subarachnoid haemorrhages. He subsequently developed a spastic paraparesis and investigations revealed a spinal angioma over the lower part of the cord. In addition, he developed chylous reflux from the scrotum due to lymphangiectasis, with incompetent valves in the lymphatic vessels connecting with the thoracic duct. Den Hartog Jager (1949) has discussed a similar case, a 27-year-old man with a spastic paraparesis due to a spinal angioma who had congenital lymphangiectasia with a chylous discharge from the right leg, and multiple cutaneous angiomas in the upper part of this limb. A case in which there was congential obstruction of the thoracic duct has also been recorded (Djindjian, Hurth and Houdart, 1970).

Vascular anomalies or tumours elsewhere in the C.N.S.

A spinal angioma has been reported in patients with a cerebral angioma (Di Chiro and Wener, 1973), cerebellar angioma (Krayenbühl, Yaşargil and McClintock, 1969) and cerebellar haemangioblastoma (Dilenge, Héon and Metzger, 1973). In one patient with bilateral retinal angiomatosis, vertebral angiography revealed the presence of at least two posterior fossa, and two cervical, angiomatous malformations (Di Chiro, 1957). In another patient with a cervical angioma supplied by the vertebral artery, there were several malformed vessels over the surface of the medulla (Kunc and Bret, 1969). In a few instances patients with a spinal angioma have been found to have an intracranial (Brion, Netsky and Zimmerman, 1952; Doppman and Di Chiro, 1965) or spinal (Herdt, Di Chiro and Doppman, 1971) arterial aneurysm.

Pia (1973) reported the coexistence of a spinal angioma and haemangioblastoma in 5 patients, but most authors do not recognise any significant association between these two lesions. This discord may relate to the diagnostic criteria employed by Pia since it is not clear from his paper whether or not the lesions were defined angiographically. In patients with a spinal intramedullary haemangioblastoma, there may be dilatation of the pial veins both above and below the tumour (Wyburn-Mason, 1943). In a minority of cases this may be so extensive that the surface of the cord is completely covered by abnormal vessels; the myelographic and operative appearances in such circumstances may resemble those of a spinal angioma, as in a case reported by Krishnan and Smith (1961). Whether these distended, tortuous pial vessels represent an associated developmental anomaly or merely a secondary effect of the tumour can only be ascertained by angiography. It may be noted, however, that the pial vessels rarely show such extensive changes in association with other spinal tumours.

A spinal angioma has also been reported in patients with an ependymoma (Vraa-Jensen, 1949; Odom, Woodhall and Margolis, 1957; Shapiro, 1968; Krieger, 1972), and in association with a spinal neurofibroma (Lombardi and Migliavacca, 1959; Shapiro, 1968). The significance of these observations is uncertain.

Other congenital anomalies

Various other congenital anomalies may be found in patients with a spinal angioma, but it is often difficult to know whether these occur more frequently than by chance. Cutaneous pigmented naevi; in either a segmental or non-segmental distribution, have been reported in a few patients (Rand, 1927; Wyburn-Mason, 1943; Ford, 1944) but this association is not specific. Similarly, non-specific vertebral abnormalities such as spina bifida occulta, and lumbarisation of the 1st sacral vertebra, may be found during radiological investigation.

Lipomas

Subcutaneous lipomas have occasionally been found in patients with either vascular malformations or haemangioblastomas of the spinal cord and its meninges (Wyburn-Mason, 1943). Since lipomas are common, such an association, which occurs only rarely, is probably of no significance.

Chapter 4
Incidence

Spinal angiomas are generally considered to be uncommon. Until recently, however, they were often not recognised unless encountered accidentally at operation, due to the diagnostic inadequacies of myelography. The development of selective spinal angiography has now permitted their direct pre-operative visualisation and, accordingly, it seems probable that they will be recognised with increasing frequency, as were their cerebral counterparts after the introduction of cerebral angiography.

The incidence of spinal angiomas is traditionally expressed as a percentage of the total number of verified spinal tumours found over the same period of time. Little more than impressions can be gleaned from the published data, which are both scanty and difficult to evaluate because they are influenced to a variable extent by case selection.

Incidence in relation to other spinal lesions

In 6 out of 130 laminectomies performed for 'spinal disease', Elsberg (1916) found no pathology other than enlarged and varicose spinal veins at the level corresponding to patients' symptoms and signs. Wyburn-Mason (1943) reviewed the early surgical literature and concluded that such abnormalities were found in 3–4 per cent of cases operated upon for spinal tumour.

However, the true nature of spinal vascular malformations may not always be recognised at operation or even at post-mortem examination, because there is probably a gradual transition between their morphological appearance and that of the normal posterior coronal veins which are themselves often large and tortuous (Kadyi, 1889). Moreover, data based solely on operative findings do not indicate the true frequency of spinal angiomas, because the natural history of these malformations may simulate conditions, such as multiple sclerosis, which do not necessitate operative treatment.

With the development and more general employment of myelography as an investigative procedure, it became possible, in some cases, to diagnose spinal angiomas pre-operatively by demonstrating the tortuous, linear filling defects which were first described by Guillain and Alajouanine (1925). Spinal angiomas are more easily visualised at myelography if large volumes of contrast material are used; in addition, the examination should be performed with the patient in the supine as well as the prone position because the majority of these malformations are located posteriorly in the lower thoracic region. An appreciation of these technical considerations has facilitated their myelographic recognition, and this has led to an increase in the relative frequency with which they are diagnosed. Thus, in the decade before 1946 only 2 cases of spinal angioma were seen at the Manchester Royal Infirmary compared with 107 cases of primary spinal tumour, while in the following decade spinal angiomas were diagnosed myelographically or at operation in 19 cases, and primary spinal tumours in 121 (Newman, 1959). In other recently published series the incidence of spinal angiomas has varied between 3·3 per cent (Krayenbühl and Yaşargil, 1963) and 11 per cent (Pia and Vogelsang, 1965) of patients with spinal tumours.

Nevertheless, studies based on the myelographic and operative diagnosis of spinal angiomas probably still under-estimate their true incidence. Thus, in the study of Teng and Papatheodorou (1964), the myelographic appearances were diagnostic in only 6 out of 12 patients with spinal vascular malformations other than telangiectasia, although the examination was always performed in both prone and supine positions, between 12 and 36 cc of contrast material being used; in the remaining patients non-specific abnormalities, sometimes inconspicuous, were found. In a larger series of 56 patients with an angiographically-defined spinal angioma, the myelographic appearances were characteristic in 48 per cent, abnormal but atypical in 42 per cent, and apparently normal in 10 per cent, although in some instances the examination was not performed satisfactorily (Djindjian, Hurth and Houdart, 1970).

Whilst the myelographic appearance may not be characteristic of an angioma, it may be sufficiently abnormal to lead to exploratory laminectomy when the diagnosis will be established. Nevertheless, it seems clear that myelographic abnormalities may sometimes be so inconspicuous that no diagnosis is made and operation is deferred. In such circumstances, patients with an angioma will be overlooked in studies on the relative frequency of these lesions.

It is important to consider whether, in some instances, lesions other than a vascular malformation may be classified erroneously as spinal angiomas on the basis of their appearance at myelography if the diagnosis is not confirmed by operation. Serpiginous myelographic filling defects are occasionally found in other conditions, but usually in association with local expansion of the cord or other abnormalities, as discussed in Chapter 11. These additional features are not typical of—but may occur with—an angioma, and the myelographic appearance in such circumstances is not usually considered to be diagnostic.

The myelographic delineation of spinal vascular malformations is inadequate because the anomalous vessels are not themselves opacified. The recent development of selective spinal angiography may lead to an increase in the frequency with which angiomas are diagnosed in patients with progressive spinal disease of obscure aetiology, but only if these patients are investigated without regard to the nature of any myelographic abnormality. The angiographic procedure, which is discussed in a later chapter, appears to be relatively safe, although clinical experience with it is still rather limited. Thus, Djindjian, Hurth and Houdart (1970) used it on 240 occasions without causing any neurological disturbance other than transient spasms of the abdomen and legs, although an allergic reaction to the contrast material caused the death of one patient; simiarly, Di Chiro and Wener (1973) found no significant deleterious effects specifically due to selective studies in their series. Accordingly, it seems unjustified to restrict the use of this technique to the investigation of patients in whom myelography has already suggested the possibility of an angioma, because other cases will continue to go unrecognised at a time when they might respond favourably to surgical treatment.

Incidence in relation to cerebral angiomas

Cerebral angiomas are diagnosed more frequently than spinal vascular malformations, but their incidence in relation to verified brain tumours is certainly not greater than the relative incidence of their spinal counterpart, ranging from 2 per cent (Olivecrona and Ladenheim, 1957) to 4 per cent (Krenchel, 1961) in different series.

The incidence of spinal angiomas in relation to cerebral ones has been reported as 1 : 4 in one series (Lombardi and Migliavacca, 1959), but more recent figures are difficult to obtain.

Incidence of asymptomatic angiomas

Patients with a spinal angioma may not develop symptoms until comparatively late in life. Accordingly, it seems probable that in some instances they may remain completely asymptomatic. As the spinal cord is usually not inspected in routine post-mortem examinations, the frequency with which this occurs cannot be established.

Chapter 5
Site, sex and age

The data presented in this chapter were derived from a personal analysis of cases previously reported individually or in small series by the authors cited in the Appendix. These earlier reports were scrutinised individually, and only those cases in which the diagnosis had been firmly established radiologically, at operation or by post-mortem examination were included in the case-material which was analysed. In many instances full clinical details had not been provided, and this restricted the number of cases available for study of particular aspects of the subject.

Although some of the points which are considered in this chapter were discussed by Aminoff and Logue (1974a) in an analysis of 60 previously unpublished cases of spinal angioma, the age distribution in that series cannot be considered a fully representative one because the majority of cases came from the National Hospitals for Nervous Diseases where a paediatric service is not provided. The only other recent series of comparable size is that of Djindjian, Hurth and Houdart (1970), but their conclusions concerning the age distribution and clinical presentation of patients differed from those of most other authors, probably as a result of case-selection; they provide a neurosurgical service and are therefore concerned especially with the investigation of patients after acute, disabling incidents such as subarachnoid haemorrhage, and with the assessment of selected patients referred from all over France for consideration of surgery rather than with the management of chronically disabled patients. Little reference has therefore been made to any individual series of cases, in order to minimise bias due to case-selection.

Site of the angioma

The location of the malformation with respect to one or other of the three arterial territories in the vertical axis of the cord is easily determined by selective spinal angiography, but many of the earlier cases were investigated prior to the introduction of this technique. In such circumstances it was usually impossible to identify the precise segmental level of the arteriovenous fistula itself, but when abnormal vessels were situated mainly or entirely in one of the three arterial territories of the cord, the shunt was assumed to lie within that region. The angioma could not be localised in this way when abnormal vessels were conspicuous in more than one of these territories, however, and such cases were therefore excluded from this part of the present study.

This may have led to a reduction in the number of mid-thoracic angiomas included in this survey, because this region is comparatively short and lies between the other two arterial territories of the cord; the venous components of mid-thoracic angiomas will therefore extend not infrequently into one or other of these adjacent territories, and such cases were deliberately excluded unless the site of the fistula had been demonstrated by angiography.

As assessed by these means, angiomas were located in the cervico-thoracic region in 17 per cent, mid-thoracic region in 11 per cent and more caudally in 72 per cent of 349 cases, while in a series of 35 cases investigated by angiography at the National Hospitals for Nervous Diseases or the Middlesex Hospital, London, the corresponding figures were 6 per cent, 11 per cent and 83 per cent (B.E.Kendall, personal communication). In contrast, Djindjian, Hurth and Houdart (1970) reported that the angioma was located in the cervical region in 12 per cent, between the 1st and 7th thoracic segments in 28 per cent and more caudally in 60 per cent of their 56 cases studied by angiography. However, the topographical division employed by them does not correspond to that of the present author, which is based on the regional blood supply to the cord and therefore in-includes the first 2 or 3 thoracic segments among the cervical. In spite of these individual differences, it is clear that most angiomas are located in the thoraco-lumbar region.

Sex distribution

GENERAL

Of 476 cases in which the sex of the patient was recorded, there were 344 males (72 per cent) and 132 females (28 per cent); in other words, males were affected approximately $2\frac{1}{2}$ times more commonly than females.

SITE OF THE ANGIOMA

In 325 instances it was possible to relate the sex of the patient to the site of the angioma. It can be seen from Table 5.1 that spinal angiomas were located in the thoraco-lumbar region in 77 per cent of male and 59 per cent of female patients; this region was, therefore, the most common site of an angioma in both sexes.

Table 5.1. Sex-related differences in the site of spinal angiomas.

	Number of cases			
	Male		Female	
Cervico-thoracic	32	(14%)	28	(30%)
Mid-thoracic	20	(9%)	10	(11%)
Thoraco-lumbar	179	(77%)	56	(59%)
Total	231		94	

The proportion of female patients with an angioma in the cervico-thoracic region was higher than the corresponding proportion of male patients. As a consequence, the sex incidence among patients with a malformation in this region was almost equal, whereas in more caudal areas there was a marked male preponderance of cases, as shown in Table 5.2.

Table 5.2. Relationship of sex incidence to location of malformation in 325 cases of spinal angioma.

	Number of cases		
	Cervico-thoracic	Mid-thoracic	Thoraco-lumbar
Males	32 (53%)	20 (67%)	179 (76%)
Females	28 (47%)	10 (33%)	56 (24%)
Total	60	30	235

The number of patients with a mid-thoracic angioma was small in both sexes but, as discussed above, the incidence of angiomas in this region may have been under-estimated.

Age distribution

GENERAL

It was possible to ascertain the age at diagnosis of 470 patients, and it ranged from less than 1 year to 75 years. The age distribution of these patients is shown in Figure 5.1, where it can be seen that in 61 per cent of cases the

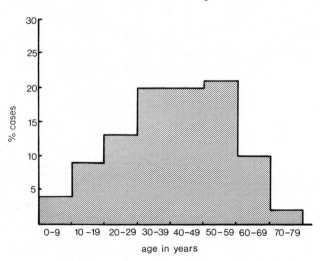

Figure 5.1. Age distribution in 470 cases at the time of diagnosis.

34   *Chapter 5*

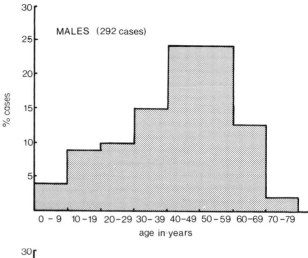

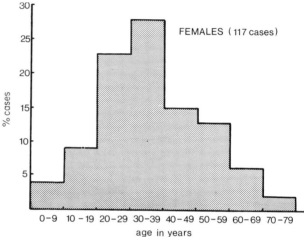

Figure 5.2. Age distribution in 292 male patients (top) and 117 females (bottom).

diagnosis was established when patients were between 30 and 59 years old. However, the male preponderance in the group of patients under consideration has undoubtedly biased these results since, as is indicated below, there are sex-related differences in the age distribution.

SEX

In 409 cases both the age and sex of the patient were provided, and this permitted the age distribution for each sex to be studied individually, as shown in Figure 5.2. It can be seen that 65 per cent of the female patients were below the age of 40 years at the time of diagnosis, compared with only 37 per cent of the males, suggesting that spinal angiomas either become symptomatic at an earlier age or lead to the development of symptoms necessitating earlier investigation in the former.

Differences in the age distribution among male and female patients could relate either to sex itself, to sex-related differences in the site of the malformation, or to both of these factors. In order to resolve this point, the age of the patient at the time of diagnosis was correlated with these two individual factors in the 311 cases for which this information was available.

The results are indicated in Table 5.3, where it can be seen that the diagnosis was usually made at a much earlier age in female patients than in males, irrespective of the angioma's site. It can also be seen, however, that in both male and female patients angiomas in the cervico-thoracic region were usually diagnosed at a much earlier age than angiomas situated elsewhere, suggesting that the location of the malformation also influenced the age distribution.

Table 5.3. Age and sex incidence in 311 cases of spinal angioma in which the location of the malformation could be related to one or other of the three main longitudinal arterial territories of the cord.

| | Cervico-thoracic | | Mid-thoracic | | Thoraco-lumbar | |
	Male	Female	Male	Female	Male	Female
Total number	34 (57%)	26 (43%)	20 (67%)	10 (33%)	169 (76%)	52 (24%)
Age-range (years)						
0–9	1 (3%)	0	1 (5%)	2 (20%)	5 (3%)	2 (4%)
10–19	7 (21%)	5 (19%)	3 (15%)	2 (20%)	12 (7%)	3 (6%)
20–29	3 (9%)	7 (27%)	0	0	10 (6%)	14 (27%)
30–39	9 (26%)	9 (35%)	3 (15%)	3 (30%)	23 (14%)	11 (21%)
40–49	7 (21%)	4 (15%)	5 (25%)	2 (20%)	43 (25%)	9 (17%)
50–59	7 (21%)	0	4 (20%)	1 (10%)	46 (28%)	7 (13%)
60–69	0	1 (4%)	3 (15%)	0	26 (15%)	4 (8%)
70–79	0	0	1 (5%)	0	4 (2%)	2 (4%)
No. diagnosed before age 40	20 (59%)	21 (81%)	7 (35%)	7 (70%)	50 (30%)	30 (58%)

Number of cases

These differences probably relate to the size of the arteriovenous shunt, and to whether or not the angioma is intramedullary, at least in part. In view of their importance these points are considered separately in the following chapter.

Summary

1 The distribution of angiomas with respect to the three arterial territories in the vertical axis of the cord, and the sex and age distribution of patients with these malformations has been studied by reference to the previously published literature.

2 Angiomas occurred most commonly in the thoraco-lumbar region in patients of either sex.

3 They occurred $2\frac{1}{2}$ times more frequently in male patients than in females. However, this male preponderance of cases did not apply to angiomas located in the cervico-thoracic region where the sex incidence was approximately equal.

4 In general, the diagnosis was usually established when patients were between 30 and 59 years of age. It was commonly established at an earlier age in female patients than males, however, irrespective of the site of the malformation. In both sexes, moreover, angiomas in the cervico-thoracic region were usually diagnosed at an earlier age than those located more caudally.

Chapter 6
The volume of
the shunt

Although spinal angiomas consist of an arteriovenous fistula, this is not always apparent when they are inspected at operation or post mortem examination, and consequently they were subdivided by earlier authors into venous and arteriovenous malformations, as discussed in Chapter 1. Their macroscopic appearance *in vivo* will depend not only upon whether the region inspected is in the vicinity of the fistula, but also upon the physical characteristics of the fistula itself. In particular, when it permits the flow of a relatively large volume of blood from arterial to venous channels, the blood contained within the veins draining a malformation will be bright red ('arterial') in colour. Similarly, the draining veins will pulsate when the anatomical and structural characteristics of the fistulous vessels permit the arterial pressure wave (pulse wave) to be propagated, and this is most likely to occur if the malformation contains a fistula of such a size and structure that a large volume of blood can flow through it.

The presence of 'arterial' blood in the veins draining a vascular malformation, and pulsation of these venous channels, suggest that a large volume of blood is flowing through the fistula, while the presence of darker blood in distended, non-pulsating, tortuous veins suggests a shunt of smaller volume. Before the advent of selective spinal angiography shunts of the latter type were often regarded as purely venous malformations on the basis of their operative appearance.

In order to determine whether the size of the shunt was of any clinical significance, the literature cited in the Appendix was scrutinised, and malformations were classified as having shunts of large or small volume depending upon their operative appearance. Cases were excluded if the information provided was insufficient to permit them being placed into one or other category.

In 224 cases it was possible to classify the malformation in this manner, and the shunt was of large volume in 105 cases (47 per cent) and small volume in 119 (53 per cent).

Sex

There were more male than female patients with shunts of either type among these 224 cases, but shunts of large volume occurred in a higher proportion of female patients (61 per cent) than males (41 per cent), as shown in Table 6.1.

Table 6.1. Sex-related differences in the volume of the shunt.		Males	Females
	Shunt of large volume	65 (41%)	40 (61%)
	Shunt of small volume	93 (59%)	26 (39%)
	Total	158	66

Location

In 154 cases it was possible to define both the volume of the shunt and the location of the malformation with respect to one or other of the three main arterial territories in the vertical axis of the spinal cord.

SHUNTS OF LARGE VOLUME

Table 6.2. Relationship of the shunt volume to the sex of the patient and location of the malformation.

It can be seen from Table 6.2 that this type of shunt occurred in 87 per cent of all the angiomas located in the cervico-thoracic region, but in a smaller proportion of malformations situated more caudally.

		Cervico-thoracic	Mid-thoracic	Thoraco-lumbar
Male and female combined	Shunt of large volume	27 (87%)	3 (33%)	53 (46%)
	Shunt of small volume	4 (13%)	6 (67%)	61 (54%)
Male	Shunt of large volume	14 (78%)	1 (17%)	38 (45%)
	Shunt of small volume	4 (22%)	5 (83%)	46 (55%)
Female	Shunt of large volume	13 (100%)	2 (67%)	15 (50%)
	Shunt of small volume	0	1 (33%)	15 (50%)

The regional distribution of malformations with this type of shunt is indicated in Table 6.3. Although the majority were in the thoraco-lumbar territory, one-third were situated in the cervico-thoracic region and a few were mid-thoracic in location.

SHUNTS OF SMALL VOLUME

Table 6.3. The regional distribution of angiomas with shunts of large and small volume.

Table 6.2 indicates that only a small proportion of cervical angiomas, but approximately half of all angiomas in the thoraco-lumbar region were of this type. The great majority of malformations with this type of shunt were located in the thoraco-lumbar region, as shown in Table 6.3.

	Shunt of large volume			Shunt of small volume		
Location of malformation	Male	Female	Male and female combined	Male	Female	Male and female combined
Cervico-thoracic	14 (26%)	13 (43%)	27 (33%)	4 (7%)	0	4 (6%)
Mid-thoracic	1 (2%)	2 (7%)	3 (3%)	5 (9%)	1 (6%)	6 (8%)
Thoraco-lumbar	38 (72%)	15 (50%)	53 (64%)	46 (84%)	15 (94%)	61 (86%)
Total	53	30	83	55	16	71

Thus, both types of shunt were located most commonly in the thoraco-lumbar territory where they occurred with a similar frequency. Shunts of small volume occurred relatively infrequently in more rostral areas in contrast to shunts of large volume which were not uncommon in the cervical region; accordingly, the majority of cervical angiomas had shunts of the latter type.

Relationship to the cord

The great majority of spinal angiomas are extramedullary in location, but some may have an intramedullary component as discussed in Chapter 10. Wyburn-Mason (1943) implied, however, that the lesion was essentially intramedullary in patients with a malformation of 'arteriovenous' type; abnormal arteries were said to run to an intramedullary mass from which abnormal veins radiated out before coursing over the surface of the cord. More recently, Djindjian, Hurth and Houdart (1970) found that a portion of the angioma was intramedullary in each of their few patients with a cervical lesion, but much less commonly in patients with a more caudal one.

These observations suggest that an intramedullary component may be present more frequently in patients with a shunt of large volume than in those with a small one, but this could not be confirmed because the evidence to support the alleged presence of an intramedullary component was inadequate in many of the previously published cases. This point, which is of considerable importance, is considered in more detail in Chapter 10, where the pathological aspects of these lesions are discussed.

Clinical relevance

AGE DISTRIBUTION

It was shown in Chapter 5 that spinal angiomas were generally diagnosed at an earlier age in female patients than males, irrespective of their location, and that cervical angiomas were usually diagnosed at an earlier age than more caudally placed malformations in patients of either sex. These differences in the age distribution are therefore similar in pattern to those described above in the relative distribution of malformations with a shunt of large volume, suggesting that patients in whom the diagnosis is established at a relatively early age usually have a shunt of this type.

In order to confirm this, the age distribution of patients with large and small shunts was compared; comparison was made between patients of the same sex and with angiomas situated within the same vertical arterial territory of the spinal cord, to prevent any bias by these factors. This so restricted the number of cases in each group, however, that no more than a general impression, which must await confirmation, could justifiably be gained. Nevertheless, the proportion of patients of each sex diagnosed before the age of 40 years was always higher among those with a shunt of large volume than those with a small one located within the same region. For example, in female patients with a thoraco-lumbar angioma the diagnosis was established before the age of 40 years in 9 (60 per cent) of the 15 with large shunts but in only 5 (33 per cent) of the 15 with small ones.

SPINAL ANGIOGRAPHY

Differences in the relative distribution of angiomas with large and small shunts are reflected by regional and age-related differences in the angiographic appearances of spinal angiomas. The presence of a large shunt can be inferred at angiography when an angioma is found to have several feeding arteries and its draining veins are rapidly opacified. These angiographic features are present in the majority of cervical angiomas but in a much lower proportion of thoraco-lumbar lesions, and are found much more commonly in children or young adults than in older patients.

SUBARACHNOID HAEMORRHAGE

This is discussed in detail in the next chapter, but it may be noted here that the incidence of subarachnoid haemorrhage from angiomas with a shunt of large volume was 25 per cent, compared with an incidence of 5 per cent from angiomas with small shunts. The volume of the shunt is therefore of considerable prognostic importance in this respect, and can often be inferred from the findings at angiography as indicated above.

Summary

1 Spinal angiomas were classified as having shunts of large or small volume depending upon their operative appearance.

2 Angiomas with large shunts occurred in a higher proportion of female patients than males, and were the most common type of malformation found in the cervical region. In the thoraco-lumbar region, shunts of large and small volume occurred with a similar frequency.

3 The volume of the shunt seemed to influence the age at which the diagnosis was established; in patients of the same sex and with malformations in the same arterial territory of the cord, the diagnosis was usually made at an earlier age when there was a large shunt.

4 These findings are reflected by regional and age-related differences in the angiographic appearances of spinal angiomas.

5 The incidence of subarachnoid haemorrhage from angiomas with a large shunt is greater than from those with small ones. The volume of the shunt is therefore of considerable prognostic importance, and can often be inferred from the findings at angiography.

Chapter 7
Spinal subarachnoid haemorrhage and haematomyelia

Spinal angiomas may give rise to two distinct types of neurological disturbance. The first, spinal subarachnoid haemorrhage, is usually dramatic in onset, is accompanied by well-defined symptoms and signs, and may have a catastrophic outcome. The second, a disturbance of function in the spinal cord and/or roots, is more variable in its mode of onset, clinical course and outcome; it is discussed in detail in the following chapter.

The diagnosis of subarachnoid haemorrhage is usually suggested by the clinical history and physical signs, and is confirmed by finding uniformly blood-stained cerebrospinal fluid at lumbar puncture. Spontaneous, or non-traumatic, spinal subarachnoid haemorrhage is far less common than the intracranial variety, occurring in less than 1 per cent of the series reported by Walton (1956). It seems likely, however, that some cases go unrecognised because they simulate an intracranial bleed, as discussed by Henson and Croft (1956).

Spinal subarachnoid haemorrhage usually occurs from one of the vessels in the subarachnoid space, or is secondary to haematomyelia with subsequent rupture of blood through the neural parenchyma and pia mater. It may also follow rupture of a subdural haematoma into the subarachnoid space, although this must be extremely uncommon. A number of pathological conditions may give rise to it, as indicated in Table 7.1, but statistics on their incidence are difficult to acquire. Spinal angiomas are probably its commonest cause, and it occurs in approximately 10 per cent of patients with these vascular anomalies. Subarachnoid haemorrhage due to other

Table 7.1. Causes of spontaneous spinal subarachnoid haemorrhage.

1 Spinal angiomas (e.g. Wyburn-Mason, 1943)

2 Other types of spinal hamartoma, e.g. telangiectases (Walton, 1956; Odom, 1962)

3 Coarctation of the aorta (Wyburn-Mason, 1943; Blackwood, 1958)

4 Rupture of a spinal artery (Hamby, 1948)

5 Mycotic and other aneurysms of a spinal artery (Henson and Croft, 1956)

6 Polyarteritis nodosa (Henson and Croft, 1956)

7 Tumours, e.g. ependymoma (Abbott, 1939; Fincher, 1951; Odom, 1962)
   neurofibroma (Krayenbühl, 1947; Fincher, 1951; Halpern, Feldman and Peyser, 1958; Prieto and Cantu, 1967; Gautier-Smith, 1967)
   'benign neuro-gliome' (André-Thomas, Ferrand, Schaeffer and De Martel, 1930)
   'neuro-spongiome' (Roger, Paillas and Duplay, 1949)
   'meningioblastome' (Roger, Paillas and Duplay, 1949)
   meningeal sarcoma (Tarlov and Keener, 1953)

8 Toxic-infective states, e.g. typhoid fever (Douglas-Wilson, Miller and Watson, 1933)
   smallpox, anthrax, septicaemia, pyaemia (Wilson, 1955)

9 Blood dyscrasias (Wilson, 1955)

10 Anticoagulant drugs (Yuhl, 1955)

causes is not considered further in the present chapter.

Since spinal subarachnoid haemorrhage is uncommon and most individual series are small, data have again been obtained by an analysis of previously published cases (the sources of which are cited in the Appendix). In this instance the large series of Djindjian, Hurth and Houdart (1970) has been excluded, however, since clinical details of individual cases were not provided.

It is of some importance to consider the criteria which were used in this study to decide whether subarachnoid haemorrhage had occurred. If proven changes in the cerebrospinal fluid, or post-mortem confirmation, are always required before accepting that it has taken place in patients with an underlying angioma, estimates of its incidence will be too low. Conversely, if any sudden exacerbation of the patient's neurological condition is attributed to it, such estimates will be deceptively high.

In this analysis a diagnosis of subarachnoid haemorrhage was accepted under one of three circumstances. First, if it had been proven by lumbar puncture or post-mortem. Second, if the author who originally reported the case had given this as the diagnosis but failed to indicate whether it had been verified; it may be assumed that in most cases confirmation was, in fact, obtained by examination of the cerebrospinal fluid, for the majority of these patients were apparently investigated in hospital by angiography to exclude an underlying intracranial vascular abnormality before the spinal origin of the bleed became apparent by subsequent developments. Finally, if the clinical manifestations of the episode in question conformed fully to those of subarachnoid haemorrhage, and both the original and the present author were satisfied that this was the probable cause of the patient's symptoms, the diagnosis was accepted even though the cerebrospinal fluid was not examined.

It should be noted that these definitive criteria are similar to, but probably more stringent than, those used in the Cooperative Study of Intracranial Aneurysms and Subarachnoid Haemorrhage, when it was generally accepted that sudden changes in neurological status indicated a bleeding episode unless due to herniation or to extracranial factors (Locksley, 1966).

Incidence

Subarachnoid haemorrhage is reported to have occurred in 53 of the 421 cases of spinal angioma which were reviewed, that is, in 12·6 per cent of cases. This is similar to the incidence of 10 per cent (6/60 cases) in the series of Aminoff and Logue (1974a), and that of 11·3 per cent reported by Newman (1959) from a review of 150 previously published cases. Although it differs from the incidence of 30 per cent cited by Djindjian and his colleagues (1969, 1970), this may well relate to case selection, for the latter authors, who provide a neurosurgical service, are probably concerned especially with the investigation and management of patients after such acute episodes, and are known to have a particular interest in spinal angiomas.

SEX

There were 25 male and 25 female patients among the 50 with subarachnoid haemorrhage whose sex was specified. However, the number of patients at risk of having a subarachnoid haemorrhage was not equal in the two sexes because spinal angiomas are more common in males than females, as shown in Chapter 5. When this was taken into account, subarachnoid haemorrhage was found to have occurred in only 8 per cent (25/306) of male patients compared to 22 per cent (25/115) of females with an underlying angioma, indicating that the risk is significantly greater among the latter.

LOCATION OF MALFORMATION

In 49 of the 53 cases of subarachnoid haemorrhage, it was possible to determine the site of the angioma with respect to one or other of the three vertical arterial territories of the spinal cord, and it was cervico-thoracic in 22, mid-thoracic in 4 and thoraco-lumbar in 23 instances. These figures were related to the total number of patients at risk from an angioma in each of these sites, in order to determine the proportion in which bleeding had occurred in each case. It was found to have occurred in 42 per cent with a cervical, 20 per cent with a mid-thoracic and 11 per cent with a thoraco-lumbar angioma, these differences being significantly greater than could have been expected by chance. The risk of subarachnoid haemorrhage is, therefore, greater in patients with a cervical angioma.

VOLUME OF THE SHUNT

In 31 of the 53 cases of subarachnoid haemorrhage it was possible to classify the underlying angioma as having a shunt of large or small volume on the basis of its operative appearance, and it was of large volume in the majority (84 per cent). The incidence of subarachnoid haemorrhage from angiomas with a shunt of large volume was 25 per cent, compared with an incidence of 5 per cent from angiomas with smaller shunts.

Further analysis of the available material showed that the higher incidence of subarachnoid haemorrhage in female patients and patients with a cervical angioma was probably related to the higher incidence of malformations with a shunt of large volume in these patients.

Age

AT DIAGNOSIS

It was possible to ascertain the age at which the underlying angioma was diagnosed in 51 of the patients who had experienced a subarachnoid haemorrhage, and it ranged from 6 to 58 years. It was not influenced by the sex of the patient or the location of the malformation. The diagnosis was made before the age of 40 years in 84 per cent of these patients, but in only 46 per cent of all patients with a spinal angioma.

AT FIRST SUBARACHNOID HAEMORRHAGE

The age of the patient at the time of his first subarachnoid haemorrhage could be determined in 50 cases, and in just over half (52 per cent) it was less than 20 years. In Table 7.2 the age distribution of these 50 patients at the

Table 7.2. The age distribution of 50 patients with a spinal angioma at the time of their first subarachnoid haemorrhage and at diagnosis.

	Age-range					
	0–9 years	10–19 years	20–29 years	30–39 years	40–49 years	50–59 years
% cases at 1st SAH	6	46	16	18	12	2
% cases at diagnosis	4	27	26	27	10	6

time of their first subarachnoid haemorrhage and at the time of diagnosis is compared. It can be seen that there was a delay in establishing the diagnosis in many patients, and this was because the spinal source of the haemorrhage was often not recognised until the later development of signs of cord dysfunction.

Clinical course

In 38 (75 per cent) of the 51 cases for which this information was available, subarachnoid haemorrhage was the first symptom produced by the underlying angioma; in the other 13 patients (25 per cent) there was a pre-existing disturbance in function of the spinal cord or nerve roots due to the angioma.

The clinical syndrome typically produced by spinal subarachnoid haemorrhage has been described by Henson and Croft (1956), Walton (1956) and Odom (1962), but it is still not widely appreciated. Haemorrhage into the spinal subarachnoid space gives rise to sudden severe pain which initially may be felt at the site of the bleeding but soon spreads to the rest of the back. There may be accompanying radicular pain, particularly in the legs where sciatica sometimes develops as blood passes into the lumbar sac. Signs of spinal meningeal irritation are usually present, consisting of spinal rigidity, head retraction and, occasionally, even opisthotonos. If the blood passes intracranially, as is likely when the source of haemorrhage is in the cervical region or the haemorrhage is profuse, there may be headache and a disturbance of consciousness which, in severe cases, may be accompanied by more widespread signs, including papilloedema, cranial nerve palsies, and convulsions. Such symptoms and signs are occasionally so prominent, and so rapid in their onset, that a mistaken diagnosis of intracranial subarachnoid haemorrhage is made. In other instances limb weakness, sensory loss, and disorders of micturition and defaecation may occur due to a disturbance of spinal cord function which results either from haematomyelia or from compression of the cord by blood or blood clot, and this usually helps to localise the source of the bleeding.

Spinal subarachnoid haemorrhage is uncommon, and consequently there is no published information concerning the gravity of the initial bleed, the frequency with which re-bleeding occurs, and the prognosis for subsequent survival in patients with an underlying angioma; accordingly, the management of such patients has depended upon clinical intuition and dogma. In order to provide a more rational basis for their future management, some of these points are considered below, but in view of the relatively small number of cases involved only tentative conclusions can be drawn.

MORTALITY FROM THE INITIAL HAEMORRHAGE

It was not possible to assess accurately the gravity of the initial haemorrhage except in the broadest of terms, because of the paucity of clinical details provided in many cases. It may be noted, however, that 3 of the 53 patients died within a few days of it.

The total number of haemorrhages known to have occurred in the 53 cases of this series is shown in Table 7.3. However, in 5 of these cases it was not possible to ascertain whether more than one episode of bleeding had occurred, because no further details were available, and 3 other patients died from their initial haemorrhage

Table 7.3. The total number of subarachnoid haemorrhages known to have occurred in the 53 cases in this series.

Number of SAHs	Number of patients
1	31
2	13
3	4
4	1
5	2
6	2
Total number of subarachnoid haemorrhages	95
Total number of patients	53

as indicated above. Accordingly, there were 45 patients who were known to be at risk of another bleed, including 4 who were operated upon at or within one month of their original haemorrhage. Twenty-two of these patients (49 per cent) had a second subarachnoid haemorrhage after an interval which varied from twenty-four hours to well over five years, and this had a fatal outcome in 4 cases. Nine (50 per cent) of the 18 survivors are known to have had 20 additional episodes of bleeding over the period of time for which further information was available. In other words, approximately half of the patients surviving the first haemorrhage had a second, and half of those surviving the second had at least one other.

The time interval between successive haemorrhages varied considerably in different patients, as can be seen from Table 7.4. In cases of multiple bleeds, there was often considerable variation in the intervals between successive episodes in the same patient.

RISK OF RE-BLEEDING AFTER THE INITIAL HAEMORRHAGE

As discussed above, re-bleeding is known to have occurred in approximately half of the patients who survived the first episode. However, this figure must be considered

Table 7.4. Interval between successive subarachnoid haemorrhages.

Time from preceding haemorrhage	2nd SAH	3rd SAH	4th SAH	5th SAH	6th SAH
Less than 1 month	4	1	1	1	
1–6 months	2	2			1
6–12 months	2				
1–2 years	3	2			
2–3 years	2	1			
3–5 years	3	1	1	1	
5–10 years	4		2	1	
Total	20	7	4	3	1

Note When a subarachnoid haemorrhage was said to have occurred at a time midway between two of the above intervals, it has been recorded under the earlier interval (e.g. a haemorrhage at 2 years is recorded under the interval 1–2 years).

Two cases have been omitted, because no information was available about re-bleeding intervals. The first had experienced 6 haemorrhages over 7 years, and the second had had 3 over 11 years.

to under-estimate the true incidence of re-bleeding, for two reasons. Firstly, there was considerable variation in the length of time after the initial bleed for which information on each patient was available. Secondly, in evaluating the information that was available, it has been assumed that a further haemorrhage did not occur unless specific reference was made to it, and this is not necessarily the case.

In order to obtain clearer insight into the risk of re-bleeding, the available data were analysed further. The number of patients who had experienced a second subarachnoid haemorrhage during successive periods of time after the initial bleed was related to the total number of patients about whom information was available, and who were known to be at risk, at the commencement of each interval. The results are summarised in Table 7.5, where the incidence of a second haemorrhage

Table 7.5. Incidence of a second subarachnoid haemorrhage at various intervals of time after the first haemorrhage.

	Time after 1st SAH						
	0–1 month	1–6 months	6–12 months	1–2 years	2–3 years	3–5 years	5+ years
No. of patients at risk of 2nd SAH	43	35	31	28	21	15	10
No. of patients having a 2nd SAH	4	2	2	3	2	3	4
No. of deaths from 2nd SAH	1			1		1	1
Incidence of 2nd SAH	9·3%	5·7%	6·5%	10·7%	9·5%	20%	40%

Note For the purpose of this table, a patient was considered at risk of a second subarachnoid haemorrhage for the length of time after the initial episode in which information about him was available, or until he re-bled, died or was operated upon.

Two cases of multiple haemorrhage have been omitted, because no information was available about re-bleeding intervals. The first had experienced 6 haemorrhages over 7 years, the second had had 3 over 11 years.

in each of these periods of time is indicated, and it can be seen that the recurrence rate within the first month was nearly 10 per cent. It can also be seen that in 8 (40 per cent) of the 20 cases of recurrent haemorrhage for which information was available, the second episode occurred within one year of the initial bleed.

MORTALITY FROM RECURRENT HAEMORRHAGE

Four of the 22 patients who had a second subarachnoid haemorrhage died as a consequence of it, and another patient died after his fifth bleeding episode. Thus 11 per cent (5/45) of the patients who survived the first bleed died from a recurrence of the haemorrhage. However, this figure should not be considered as more than a conservative guide to the actual mortality rate from recurrent haemorrhage among such patients, because 4 of the cases in this series were operated upon within a month of the initial bleed and the subsequent medical status of the others was documented for only a limited and variable period. It is of value, nevertheless, in indicating the lower limit of the mortality rate that can be anticipated.

FACTORS INFLUENCING THE DEVELOPMENT OF SUBARACHNOID HAEMORRHAGE

It seemed unlikely that the development of subarachnoid haemorrhage was related to systemic hypertension in view of the age distribution of affected patients, and this was confirmed by examination of the available data. In 2 cases it might have been related to preceding trauma, and in 2 other cases there was a history that trauma, of dubious significance, had occurred some time previously.

It was not possible to determine whether there was any association between the size of the angioma and the development of subarachnoid haemorrhage, because of the paucity of available data. Herdt, Di Chiro and Doppman (1971) found that subarachnoid haemorrhage had occurred in 3 of their 50 cases of spinal angioma, in each of which there was a coexisting saccular arterial aneurysm, and they were able to cite 4 similar cases from the literature. The present author, reviewing these other cases, found that in one there was merely an irregular distension of the fistulous portion of the angioma, and in another subarachnoid haemorrhage had not occurred, although pathological study did reveal evidence of previous intramedullary bleeding. Nevertheless, it may well be that there is a greater risk of subarachnoid haemorrhage among the rare patients in whom a spinal arterial aneurysm coexists with the angioma.

It has been shown that half of the patients with an underlying spinal angioma who survived one subarachnoid haemorrhage had at least one other. Study of the available clinical material revealed no specific factor, common to these cases of recurrent haemorrhage, which might provide a guide to prognosis after the initial bleed. In particular, there was no significant association between either the age or sex of the patient, or the site of the malformation, and recurrence of the episode.

OVERALL MORTALITY RATE

Eight patients died as a result of subarachnoid haemorrhage, making a mortality rate of 15 per cent in the 53 cases of spinal angioma that had bled. Again, however, this figure must be considered as a conservative estimate for the reasons discussed above.

There were 421 cases of spinal angioma which were reviewed originally, and of these 53 are known to have had one or more subarachnoid haemorrhages which resulted in 8 deaths. The mortality rate from subarachnoid haemorrhage in patients with a spinal angioma is, therefore, at least 1·9 per cent.

HAEMATOMYELIA

It was difficult to decide on clinical grounds alone whether haematomyelia was associated with the subarachnoid haemorrhage, because spinal cord dysfunction may result from compression by blood or blood clot. In the majority of cases, conspicuous signs of cord dysfunction did not accompany the haemorrhage, although in many they developed at a later date as part of the progressive myelopathy which may occur in patients with a spinal angioma. In 7 cases, however, post-mortem examination indicated that haematomyelia had occurred, and the clinical signs in 6 of the surviving patients were very suggestive of this.

Management

DIAGNOSIS

Clinical assessment suggests the diagnosis of subarachnoid haemorrhage, and this is confirmed by examination of the cerebrospinal fluid. It may be difficult to recognise the spinal origin of the haemorrhage, however, unless the clinical features are characteristic, there are signs of cord or root dysfunction, or a bruit is audible over the spine. For this reason, many patients in this series were initially investigated by carotid and vertebral angiography in order to visualise an intracranial source of the bleeding. Once its spinal origin has become apparent, myelography should be performed to establish the underlying cause, but this is usually delayed until the cerebrospinal fluid is clear of blood unless there are signs of increasing cord dysfunction.

If the myelographic appearance is suggestive of an angioma and surgical treatment is contemplated, selective spinal angiography must be undertaken to define its feeding and draining vessels, the site of the fistula, and the local source of supply to the anterior spinal artery. Exploratory laminectomy is usually indicated when the myelogram suggests the presence of an intradural tumour. If myelography fails to reveal an underlying cause, and there is no evidence of inflammatory, infective or haematological disorder, selective spinal angiography may achieve the delineation of an otherwise inconspicuous vascular anomaly.

TREATMENT

By analogy with the management of intracranial subarachnoid haemorrhage, it seems reasonable to keep patients in bed for 4 weeks or so, in order to avoid physical exertion which might precipitate a further haemorrhage. Analgesics should be given as necessary for the relief of pain, and meticulous care of the skin, bladder and bowels may be required if there is a derangement of cord function. As discussed in Chapter 12, the treatment of choice for the underlying angioma is its surgical excision, or the intradural ligation of its feeding vessels, in order to prevent recurrence of the haemorrhage or the later development of other neurological disturbances. This must sometimes be delayed, however, if the available angiographic and surgical facilities are restricted, and may even be contra-indicated if the angioma is intramedullary or is intimately connected with the intramedullary circulation. In such circumstances, decompressive laminectomy, with evacuation of subarachnoid clot, may be necessary if there is clinical and myelographic evidence of spinal cord compression; alternatively, systemic steroid therapy may be helpful if there are signs of increasing cord dysfunction without evidence of extramedullary compression.

Summary

1 Spinal angiomas are probably the commonest cause of spinal subarachnoid haemorrhage.

2 Subarachnoid haemorrhage occurred in 12·6 per cent of previously published cases of spinal angioma. In the majority of these, it occurred from an angioma with a shunt of large volume. There was a higher incidence of subarachnoid haemorrhage in female patients than males, and in patients with a cervical angioma than those with a more caudally situated lesion, due probably to the higher incidence of angiomas with a shunt of large volume in these patients.

3 Over half of the angiomas that bled had done so at least once before patients were 20 years old, and in the majority of cases this was the first manifestation of the underlying malformation. However, the spinal source of the haemorrhage was often not recognised until the later development of signs of cord dysfunction.

4 The syndrome of spinal subarachnoid haemorrhage consists typically of symptoms and signs of spinal meningeal irritation, which may be accompanied by a disturbance in function of the spinal cord or roots. Cerebral symptoms may also occur if the blood passes rostrally.

5 Approximately half of the patients who survived the first haemorrhage had a second, and half of the subsequent survivors had further bleeding episodes. The second bleed occurred within one year of the initial episode in 40 per cent of the cases with recurrent haemorrhage. It was not possible to recognise any specific factors which provided a guide to prognosis after the initial bleed.

6 The overall mortality rate from subarachnoid haemorrhage was 15 per cent in the 53 cases of spinal angioma that had bled, and 1·9 per cent in the entire series. Due to the manner in which the data were obtained, these figures probably under-estimate the true figures.

7 The management of patients with haemorrhage from an underlying angioma is discussed. Detailed radiological studies are necessary to define the malformation which should be treated by surgical excision or ligation of feeding vessels, when feasible.

Chapter 8
Clinical
features
of spinal
angiomas

The clinical features of spinal angiomas have received relatively little attention in the past. Although Wyburn-Mason (1943) discussed them in his monograph, he provided detailed case histories of his patients rather than a comprehensive analysis of their symptoms and signs, and most of the other accounts deal only with restricted aspects of the subject or with small series of cases. The present account is therefore based to a large extent on a recent study (Aminoff and Logue, 1974a, b) of the medical records of 60 cases, most of which were from the National Hospitals for Nervous Diseases. The diagnosis was established by myelography in 53 of these cases, and in 31 it was subsequently confirmed by angiography or direct inspection; in the remaining 7 cases myelography was either not performed or was not diagnostic, and the angioma was found at exploratory laminectomy or post-mortem examination.

Symptoms and signs

The series consisted of 48 male and 12 female patients. They ranged in age between 21 and 75 years, but the majority (49 patients) were more than 40 years old at the time of diagnosis. Presenting symptoms commenced insidiously in 48 cases (80 per cent) and acutely in 12 (20 per cent), usually progressing until patients were left with some degree of permanent disability. Although the precise segmental level of the angioma had not always been determined, it was below the mid-thoracic region of the cord in at least two-thirds of cases, as in most other series. Disturbances in the legs and trunk, and in the control of micturition, defaecation and sexual function were therefore the usual clinical manifestations of the underlying lesion.

The initial symptoms of these malformations and those present at the time of diagnosis are indicated in Table 8.1, while patients' motor and sensory signs are summarised in Table 8.2.

MOTOR

Symptoms

Weakness of the legs was the initial symptom in about one-third of cases, but by the time of diagnosis it was present in almost all patients. The severity of weakness sometimes fluctuated from day to day, and was often enhanced by exercise or certain postures. In some instances it progressed with great rapidity so that patients

Table 8.1. Symptoms in 60 patients.

	Number of patients	
	Initial symptoms	Symptoms when diagnosed
Pain	25	49
Weakness	19	57
Sensory disturbance	20	52
Disturbed micturition	4	56
Disturbed defaecation	1	39
Disturbed sexual function	1	10
Subarachnoid haemorrhage	3	6

were confined to bed within a few months, but in other cases it remained mild, causing little functional disability for many years, as discussed in Chapter 9. When the malformation involved the cervical or upper thoracic region, weakness and clumsiness sometimes occurred also in the upper limbs.

Table 8.2. Motor and sensory signs in 60 patients when diagnosed.

	Number of patients	
	With sensory deficit*	Without sensory deficit
Motor signs		
Mixed upper and lower motor neurone	31	1
Lower motor neurone	14	3
Upper motor neurone	9	1
No signs	0	1
Total	54	6

* The sensory deficit was radicular in 2 patients, both of whom had a mixed upper and lower motor neurone disturbance, and was more extensive in the other 54 patients.

Signs

In early stages there was frequently some variability of motor signs and there was sometimes no detectable weakness even when the patient was re-examined after exercise. Examination at a later stage revealed that weakness was usually generalised and there was often associated muscle wasting, particularly about the thighs and buttocks. In many instances, however, there were coexisting signs which traditionally are associated with an upper motor neurone lesion, and in 14 cases the weakness itself had a 'pyramidal' distribution in the legs, affecting the flexor muscles to a greater extent than the extensors.

The plantar responses were extensor on one or both sides in 38 cases at the time of diagnosis, being flexor or unobtainable in roughly equal proportions among the remaining patients. Some abnormality of the tendon reflexes was usually found, either a diminution (32 cases), an increase (18 cases), or a combination of these changes (8 cases). In one-third of cases an extensor plantar response was found in association with absence of at least one of the tendon reflexes in the legs, emphasising the mixed nature of the motor deficit in many patients.

The pattern of motor signs in the legs at the time of diagnosis was indicative of a 'pyramidal' disturbance in 10 cases, a lower motor neurone lesion in 17, and a combined disturbance in 32, the remaining patient having no motor signs whatsoever.

In patients with a cervical angioma, weakness in the arms was usually—but not always—of a predominantly lower motor neurone type.

SENSORY

Symptoms

Pain was the initial symptom of the angioma in about 40 per cent of cases, but by the time of diagnosis more than 80 per cent of patients complained of it, as shown in Table 8.1. The distribution of this pain is indicated in Table 8.3. In the majority of cases it was either

Table 8.3. Distribution of pain and other sensory symptoms at the time of diagnosis.

	Distribution	Number of patients
Pain (49 patients)	Back and radicular	15
	Back only	13
	Radicular only	11
	Back and diffuse	4
	Diffuse only	3
	Back, radicular and diffuse	2
	Radicular and diffuse	1
Other sensory symptoms (52 patients)	Diffuse only	36
	Radicular only	10
	Radicular and diffuse	6

Note 'Diffuse' is used to designate symptoms occurring in the limbs in a non-radicular distribution.

localised to the back as dull ache, confined to a radicular distribution usually in the limbs but sometimes in the trunk, or occurred in both of these situations. Less commonly, diffuse non-segmental pain was felt, either alone or in combination with the other varieties described above, in the periphery of a limb. Limb pain, whether radicular or non-segmental in distribution, frequently occurred intermittently, was burning or sharp in character, and was enhanced by exercise or certain postures. Pain sometimes preceded other symptoms by many years, and was often attributed erroneously to a prolapsed intervertebral disc.

Sensory symptoms other than pain occurred as an

initial symptom in one-third of cases, and again were much more common by the time of diagnosis (Table 8.1). Their distribution was sometimes radicular but usually was more extensive, as shown in Table 8.3, due presumably to a disturbance of cord function or involvement of multiple nerve roots. Tingling, numbness, dysaesthesiae, hyperpathia or a feeling of constriction frequently commenced in an extremity, extending later to the trunk and perineum.

Signs

In a few patients, examination at an early stage revealed no abnormality other than hyperpathia in the distribution of their sensory symptoms, but signs were usually more widespread by the time that patients were referred to hospital. They were often patchy in distribution and sometimes varied in severity from day to day, but proprioceptive loss was occasionally so marked that gait was grossly ataxic.

An upper level of the sensory deficit was frequently found on the abdomen, but this was usually poorly defined and extended over several segments with, in some cases, a zone of hyperpathia immediately above it. The sensory level did not always correlate well with the site of the arteriovenous shunt as defined by angiography, nor with the myelographic abnormalities which were often extensive.

A partial Brown-Séquard syndrome was found in 3 patients with an acute exacerbation or onset of symptoms, and this was helpful in indicating the spinal origin of their disability.

At the time of diagnosis, sensory changes were absent in 6 of the 60 cases in this series, were confined to a radicular distribution in 2, and were more extensive in the remaining 52 patients, the majority of whom had impairment of both cutaneous and deep sensibility. In 12 patients there was a dissociated sensory loss, with relative preservation of light touch appreciation in the legs, and partial sacral sparing was found in 7 cases.

THE CUTANEOUS ABDOMINAL REFLEXES

In 41 of the 57 cases in which observations were recorded, these reflexes were diminished or unobtainable in one or both of the lower abdominal quadrants, and often in the upper ones as well. This presumably related either to involvement of the reflex arcs which traverse the lower six segments of the thoracic cord, or to a functional disturbance of descending corticospinal pathways.

MICTURITION, DEFAECATION AND SEXUAL FUNCTION

Although relatively infrequent initially, a disturbance of micturition was present in 56 of the 60 patients by the time of diagnosis, and was sometimes accompanied by disturbances of defaecation and sexual function. Hesitancy, often with intermittent retention, was the most frequent complaint (34 cases), but urgency was also common (19 cases), and both of these symptoms were sometimes troublesome in the same patient at different times. Other symptoms which occurred included total incontinence (10 cases), stress incontinence (2 cases), terminal dribbling (5 cases), and impaired sensation from the bladder or urethra (8 and 13 cases respectively).

Urinary symptoms were occasionally severely disabling from their onset, and sometimes occurred at a time when somatic symptoms were still relatively inconspicuous. Thus, total urinary incontinence was the first indication of any disturbance in the control of micturition in 6 (10 per cent) of the present cases.

In 39 patients there was an accompanying disturbance of defaecation, which commenced with constipation in 31, incontinence in 7 and an impaired sensation of rectal fullness in 2 (in 1 of whom it was associated with constipation). Symptoms often increased in severity with time, so that by the time of diagnosis 13 patients were or had been incontinent, and 16 had a disturbance of the sensation normally associated with defaecation, but the precise nature of this sensory disturbance was not always clear from the available records. In several instances, examination revealed that the anus was patulous and the anal reflex was lost.

Impotence was apparently rare as an initial manifestation of the underlying angioma, but it was difficult to assess its true incidence because comment about sexual function had frequently been omitted from the history. In the present series at least 10 of the 48 male patients were known to have had some disturbance of sexual function by the time of diagnosis, and the true figure was probably higher.

SPINAL SUBARACHNOID HAEMORRHAGE

This was discussed in detail in the previous chapter where it was emphasised that, in general, subarachnoid haemorrhage has a higher incidence in female patients than males, and in patients with a cervical angioma than those with a more caudally situated lesion. In the present series it was the initial manifestation of the underlying angioma in 3 patients, and by the time of diagnosis it had occurred in 6 (10 per cent), of whom 2 were female. The angioma was located in the cervical region in 2 cases and in the thoraco-lumbar region in 3; the remaining patient had a thoracic angioma but its level had not been determined more precisely. Recurrent haemorrhage occurred in one case, but its source was not identified until the later development of signs indicating a disturbance of function in the spinal cord. This case is summarised below and discussed in detail in the Appendix (p. 165).

A Jamaican tax-collector, aged 58 years, was admitted to the Maida Vale Hospital (65485) with a 7-month history of left-sided weakness. He had experienced 6 subarachnoid haemorrhages in the previous 17 years, but carotid and vertebral angiography, performed elsewhere on 2 occasions, showed no abnormality. Examination revealed a partial Brown-Séquard syndrome and myoclonic jerking of the left abductor pollicis brevis muscle. Myelography and subclavian angiography revealed a spinal angioma in the cervical region.

SPINAL BRUIT

The presence of a spinal or paraspinal bruit is of considerable diagnostic significance. The first report of such a bruit over the site of an angioma is probably that of Höök and Lidvall (1958), and the importance of auscultation over the spine was subsequently emphasised by Matthews (1959) who reported 2 further cases. Many of the other published accounts of patients with a spinal angioma fail even to refer to auscultation, and it is probable that this simple clinical procedure is still frequently overlooked when patients with a subarachnoid haemorrhage or myelopathy of uncertain aetiology are being assessed. In only 12 of the present cases was it known with certainty that auscultation over the spine had been performed, and in 2 a bruit was present.

Spinal deformities, such as kyphosis and scoliosis, were occasionally found, but are of little diagnostic significance.

As discussed in Chapter 3, a cutaneous angioma may be present and, when situated over the trunk, may receive its blood supply from the same segmental source as the spinal lesion. The presence of a cutaneous angioma may thus suggest the possibility of a spinal one in patients with cord dysfunction of obscure aetiology. However, the sites of the two lesions may be topographically unrelated, and cutaneous angiomas may also occur in association with other types of spinal hamartoma, and with epidural or vertebral angiomas.

Only 2 of the patients in this series had a cutaneous angioma, and in neither was it related to the segmental level of the spinal lesion.

COMBINATION OF SYMPTOMS AND SIGNS

By the time of diagnosis, 65 per cent of patients complained of weak legs, disturbed control of micturition, sensory symptoms and pain, while in the remainder two or more of these symptoms were present. Examination revealed a motor and sensory deficit in the legs in 90 per cent of cases; the motor deficit consisted of an upper or lower motor neurone disturbance in 40 per cent, and a combined disturbance in 50 per cent, while the sensory changes were due to a derangement in function of the cord or of multiple nerve roots in almost all cases. The remaining 10 per cent of patients had signs of a motor disturbance only, or more rarely no deficit whatsoever (Table 8.2). Although no patient in this series had sensory signs without an accompanying motor disturbance at the time of diagnosis, such cases have been recorded by others.

As might have been anticipated, weakness and sensory changes occurred also in the upper limbs when the angioma was situated in the cervical or upper thoracic region.

In general terms, therefore, the individual symptoms and signs were similar to those caused by any localised lesion, but there was evidence in most patients that the resulting disturbance of function was extensive in both longitudinal and transverse axes of the spinal cord. The presence, in addition, of a cutaneous angioma or spinal bruit should always suggest the possibility of an underlying angioma in patients with myelopathy and/or radiculopathy of obscure aetiology. Similarly, some aspects of the history, which are discussed in the following section, may also be suggestive of this.

Some aspects of the natural history

A number of factors appeared to provoke or exacerbate symptoms in some of the cases studied, and these are considered in detail below. Such associations have been commented upon by other authors, and reference is made to these earlier cases when appropriate. Any discussion about the basis of these associations, and further reference to the mode of onset and progression of symptoms have been postponed to Chapter 10, however, where they are correlated with the underlying pathology.

TRAUMA

Patients sometimes related their symptoms to previous trauma, and the validity of such an association, which may have medico-legal implications, is difficult to ascertain. On the one hand, the onset of symptoms may not be appreciated until it is brought to the patient's attention by the injury, and previously unrecognised disability may even have led to the injury. Moreover, about 5 per cent of patients in general medical and surgical wards are able to recall an injury sustained within three months of the onset of their disease (McAlpine and Compston, 1952). On the other hand, an injury may be discounted by patients with an angioma, particularly when it involves a part of the body remote from the site of symptoms.

Insufficient information is available to permit this point to be resolved satisfactorily. Nevertheless, symptoms of spinal cord dysfunction due to an underlying angioma commenced or advanced abruptly within a few days of preceding trauma in 5 cases in this series, and clinical impression suggests that disability might have been postponed but for the injury. Such a temporal relationship of symptoms to injury has been noted by many other authors, including Sargent (1925), Fine (1961), and Strain (1964). It is illustrated particularly well by the following case, originally reported by Rand (1927).

> A violinist, aged 30 years, with a three year history of slowly progressive weakness in the left leg, fell during a game of baseball. Within 48 hours he became paraplegic and lost all control of micturition and defaecation. On examination, he had a virtually complete flaccid paraplegia, with anaesthesia to the level of the 2nd lumbar dermatome. Laminectomy revealed a spinal angioma, and one of its exposed vessels was seen to be thrombosed.

Symptoms were precipitated by exercise and relieved by rest in 19 of the 60 cases which were studied, and such an association has been noted previously (e.g. Wyburn-Mason, 1943). Pain was the symptom most commonly produced, and this was either localised to the back or legs, or occurred in both situations. When felt in the legs, it was usually radicular in distribution but simulated pain due to peripheral vascular disease in its relationship to exercise. In some patients pain was the only symptom produced, but in others weakness and/or dysaesthesiae occurred in one or both legs, with or without associated pain. Motor and sensory symptoms often involved the entire limb from their onset, but in other cases they were more localised initially, sometimes extending further if exercise was continued.

The amount of exercise necessary to produce symptoms varied considerably in different patients, and usually lessened with time in individual cases so that exercise tolerance diminished. In almost all cases symptoms remitted after no more than a few minutes' rest, only to recur after a variable period when exercise was resumed. This is illustrated by the following case which has recently come to the author's attention and is reported here with the kind permission of Mr J. Andrew FRCS.

A retired civil servant, aged 60 years, gave a 15 month history of paraesthesiae in both feet. Three months after their onset he was walking up a hill when he developed weakness of such severity in the legs that he fell to the ground and was not immediately able to rise again. After resting for 2 minutes, however, he was able to get up and continue his walk. This recurred on several occasions, and his exercise tolerance gradually diminished. Eventually he could not even walk about the house for more than a few yards without collapsing to the floor, unable to get up until he had rested for 3 or 4 minutes. Initial examination revealed sensory impairment in both legs, but no motor deficit whatsoever; after exercise, however, the hip flexor and knee extensor muscles were weak bilaterally. He was admitted to the Middlesex Hospital (R 20637) where myelography and spinal angiography demonstrated an angioma in the lower thoracic region. The malformation was supplied by the 9th right intercostal artery which was clipped intradurally.

Symptoms, particularly pain, were sometimes related to a specific posture which varied in different patients. This association occurred in 14 patients in this series, and has been recorded previously by others (e.g. Wyburn-Mason, 1943; Odom, Woodhall and Margolis, 1957). Symptoms were induced or exacerbated by sitting, standing or stooping forward, and were rapidly relieved by changing to a different position, as in the following case.

> An engineer, aged 53 years, was admitted to the National Hospital (A 35108) complaining of painful paraesthesiae in the buttocks and legs which occurred when he was sitting and were relieved by standing. He had also developed hesitancy of micturition, constipation, loss of rectal sensation, and a variable weakness in the legs which was aggravated by bending forward. Myelography demonstrated a spinal angioma which was excised. Further details are given in the Appendix (p. 147).

In several of the previously published cases symptoms were related to lying flat (Wyburn-Mason, 1943) and were thus particularly troublesome at night.

PREGNANCY

Cases in which pregnancy appeared to aggravate or precipitate symptoms have been described by several authors including Delmas-Marsalat (1941), Brion, Netsky and Zimmerman (1952), Girarde and Garde (1955), Newman (1958), Fine (1961), and Schott, Cotte, Trillet and Bady (1963), and similar association has also been recorded in patients with a vertebral or extradural angioma. In some instances the symptoms evoked were catastrophically disabling and failed to resolve at the conclusion of the pregnancy.

In only one patient in the present series did symptoms show any relationship to pregnancy:

> A housewife, aged 33 years, had experienced severe left-sided sciatica in each of her three pregnancies over the preceding 10 years. She was admitted to the National Hospital (A 59239) with leg weakness and urinary retention of acute onset. Myelography suggested the presence of a spinal angioma which was confirmed by angiography. Further details are given in the Appendix (p. 155).

Insufficient information is available from the literature to permit any assessment of the risk that pregnancy will lead to onset or relapse of symptoms.

MENSTRUAL CYCLE

In rare instances symptoms have been related to menstruation, as in cases reported by Pappenheim (1938) and Epstein, Beller and Cohen (1949). The former is of particular interest.

A woman, aged 30 years, was well until the commencement of her menstrual period when she developed numbness in the left foot, which rapidly spread to the rest of the body but cleared 'in a short time'. At the end of her period, however, she developed paraesthesiae, numbness and weakness in all limbs, retention of urine and shortness of breath. She recalled having experienced similar episodes of transient heaviness of the limbs during her mentrual periods in previous years. She was admitted to hospital and found to have signs of meningeal irritation and a lesion in the cervical cord, and blood in the cerebrospinal fluid. She died soon after, and post-mortem examination revealed a cervical angioma with intramedullary and subarachnoid haemorrhage.

INFECTION OR INCREASE IN BODY TEMPERATURE

A non-specific infective illness preceded the onset or advance of symptoms in 3 of the patients in this series, and in cases reported by Brion, Netsky and Zimmerman (1952) and Nielsen, Marvin and Seletz (1958). This may have related to an associated change in body temperature, for a temporary aggravation of symptoms also occurred in 2 patients when they were taking a hot bath. Such a phenomenon is well recognised to occur in other neurological disorders, and particularly in multiple sclerosis.

OTHER FACTORS

In one patient in this series an acute exacerbation of symptoms was related to the intramuscular administration of corticotrophin (ACTH).

An industrial radiologist, aged 50 years, was admitted to his local hospital with pain, weakness and sensory symptoms in the legs. Examination revealed a spastic paraparesis, a diagnosis of multiple sclerosis was made, and a course of intramuscular ACTH prescribed. Four hours after the first injection he developed profound weakness and numbness in the legs, where the tendon reflexes could not be elicited. He recovered over the following 24 hours, but a similar exacerbation occurred 3 days later when ACTH was given again. He was transferred to the National Hospital (A 67666) where myelography and spinal angiography demonstrated an angioma. Further details are given in the Appendix (p. 153).

Two patients in this series found that leg weakness was exacerbated by straining at stool, and Therkelsen (1958) reported a patient with symptoms that initially were related to breath holding; this may relate to increased venous engorgement of the underlying malformation in such circumstances.

Cerebrospinal fluid

In the present series, manometric evidence of obstruction in the subarachnoid space was found in only one of the 17 patients in whom the response to Queckenstedt's manoeuvre had been recorded.

The cerebrospinal fluid was abnormal in 38 (76 per cent) of the 50 patients without subarachnoid haemorrhage for whom full information was available, as shown in Table 8.4. The protein content was more than 50 mg per cent in 35 of these cases, the highest value being

Table 8.4. Analysis of cerebrospinal fluid in 50 patients.*

Protein content (mg per cent)	Number of cases	Case with associated pleocytosis
0– 50	15	3
51– 75	8	1
76–100	11	1
101–150	11	5
151–200	3	0
201–300	1	1
501–600	1	0
Total	50	11

* Patients with subarachnoid haemorrhage have been excluded.

520 mg per cent, while the white cell count was increased, ranging from 6 to 50 cells per cu mm, in 11 cases, in 3 of which this was the sole abnormality. In 4 patients with a pleocytosis, the fluid had been examined soon after an acute episode.

These observations therefore accord well with those of Wyburn-Mason (1943) and Djindjian, Houdart and

Hurth (1969) who also found that subarachnoid obstruction was uncommon, that the protein content of the cerebrospinal fluid was often elevated, in a few cases to over 1000 mg per cent, and that a pleocytosis was sometimes related to an acute neurological incident.

The cerebrospinal fluid was completely normal in 24 per cent of the present cases and in 20 per cent of those in the similar series of Djindjian, Houdart and Hurth (1969).

Differential diagnosis

The early diagnosis of spinal angiomas is of considerable importance because the extent of recovery after surgical treatment of the underlying lesion depends in part upon the degree of incapacity at the time of operation. Symptoms may commence either insidiously or abruptly, and progress steadily or episodically until there is severe disability, as discussed in the following chapter. They may relate to a disturbance of function in the spinal cord and/or one or more nerve roots, and are often mistakenly attributed to some of the more common neurological disorders which are briefly discussed below.

SPINAL CORD COMPRESSION

Clinical evidence of a single progressive lesion usually indicates the need for myelography. Preliminary clinical distinction between an intramedullary tumour or extramedullary compressive lesion and a spinal angioma is often impossible. An acute onset of symptoms, their episodic progression with periods of partial remission, and their relationship to exercise, posture or other precipitating factors suggests the possibility of an angioma, however, as does the presence of a spinal bruit or signs indicating an extensive lesion in the longitudinal axis of the cord.

LUMBAR DISC LESION

This may be simulated when there is a history of radicular and back pain, but in patients with an angioma signs are usually widespread, indicating extensive involvement of the cord and roots, and Lasegue's sign (restriction by pain of passive straight-leg raising) is rarely found.

MULTIPLE SCLEROSIS

In the spinal form of this disease the history may closely resemble that of patients with a spinal angioma, but pain is usually a less prominent feature, signs of lower motor neurone involvement are inconspicuous or absent, and there may be some abnormality of the cranial nerves. In patients with progressive disability from a single cord lesion, myelography should always be undertaken before a provisional diagnosis of multiple sclerosis is made unless clinical examination, or a delayed evoked response to retinal stimulation by pattern reversal, indicates that function in other parts of the central nervous system is also disturbed.

OTHER DISORDERS

Motor neurone disease may be simulated when sensory disturbances are slight, but conspicuous disturbances of micturition and restriction of signs to the lower part of the body will indicate the need for further investigation.

Subacute combined degeneration of the cord may produce signs which are confined to the lower limbs and resemble those found in patients with a spinal angioma, but disturbances of micturition seldom occur early in this disease, there may be evidence of coexisting anaemia, and the serum B_{12} level is low.

Acute spinal poliomyelitis is occasionally diagnosed in patients who are subsequently found to have an angioma, but the presence in most cases of pyramidal signs, sensory loss or sphincter disturbance should prevent such confusion.

Acute transverse or ascending myelitis cannot be distinguished with certainty from the myelopathy which sometimes develops abruptly in patients with a spinal angioma, except by myelography. Meningo-vascular syphilis may produce a similar clinical disturbance, but there may be accompanying pupillary changes, and serological tests on blood and cerebrospinal fluid are usually positive.

Summary

1 Spinal angiomas are usually related to the lower part of the cord, and accordingly they lead most commonly to motor and sensory disturbances in the legs, and to disorders of micturition, defaecation and sexual function. Further conclusions about the clinical features of these malformations are based on an analysis of the medical records of 60 cases.

2 The most common initial symptoms were pain (42 per cent), other sensory symptoms (33 per cent), and

weakness (32 percent), and one or more of these symptoms was the initial manifestation of the underlying angioma in 85 per cent of cases, sometimes in association with other symptoms. A disturbance of micturition, defaecation or sexual function was the initial symptom in 10 per cent, and subarachnoid haemorrhage occurred in 5 per cent.

3 Symptoms were usually progressive, and by the time of diagnosis 65 per cent of patients complained of weakness, sensory symptoms, pain and disturbances of micturition; in the remainder, two or more of these symptoms were present. The incidence of subarachnoid haemorrhage had also increased to 10 per cent by this time. Examination revealed that almost all patients had motor signs in the legs; these were indicative either of an isolated upper or lower motor neurone disturbance, or more commonly of a mixed disturbance. Sensory deficits were usually extensive, but occasionally were confined to a radicular distribution. In 90 per cent of cases, both motor and sensory signs were present in the legs, while in rare cases there was no deficit whatsoever. In patients with a cervical angioma, symptoms and signs were sometimes present also in the arms. A bruit was audible over the spine in 2 cases, and a cutaneous angioma was present in 2 other patients.

4 Symptoms were precipitated or aggravated by trauma, exercise, posture, systemic infection or an increase in body temperature in several cases, by pregnancy in one, intramuscularly administered corticotrophin in another, and by straining at stool in 2. Other authors have noted also an association with the menstrual cycle, and with breath holding.

5 The cerebrospinal fluid was abnormal in 76 per cent of cases; there was usually an elevated protein content, with or without an associated pleocytosis, but in some instances an increased cell content was the sole abnormality.

6 The clinical diagnosis of spinal angiomas depends, firstly, on an accurate history and, secondly, on the presence of signs indicating an extensive lesion in the longitudinal axis of the spinal cord. A spinal bruit or cutaneous angioma, when present, provides strong support for such a diagnosis. The distinction of these malformations from other, more common neurological disorders is briefly discussed.

Chapter 9
Further
aspects of the
natural history

Scrutiny of previously published accounts provides information of only limited value concerning the natural history of spinal angiomas because most earlier authors have used descriptive but undefined terms which make it difficult to compare individual series of cases. There are, for example, divergent opinions about the meaning of the word 'remission', which seems to be used to refer either to a complete clearing of symptoms, to any temporary improvement of symptoms, however slight, or to periods in which symptoms cease to progress in severity. Similarly, the distinction between an abrupt and an insidious onset of symptoms is rarely made clear, while the time for which any temporary aggravation of symptoms must persist before it is classed as a distinct neurological 'episode' seems to depend on personal intuition rather than strictly defined criteria. Finally, there is no general agreement about the most satisfactory manner in which to grade the severity of symptoms or the progression of disability.

The clinical course of patients with these malformations, and the prognosis with regard to disability have therefore been studied (Aminoff and Logue, 1974a, b) by reference to the medical records of the 60 cases previously described in Chapter 8, and the conclusions reached are briefly contrasted with those of other authors.

Definitions

For the purpose of this discussion the following descriptive terms have been used as indicated below. Some of these definitions depend in part on subjective criteria, but this is unavoidable in clinical practice and does not necessarily detract from any practical value that they may have.

Acute and insidious onset of symptoms

These terms refer both to the severity of the first symptoms of the angioma and to the rate at which they develop When they immediately cause distress or functional disability, or advance to this extent within 24 hours, they are described as acute in onset; because of their severity, patients can often recall with accuracy the time that they commenced. The onset is described as insidious when symptoms do not reach this degree of severity within 24 hours, and in such circumstances their precise time of onset is usually not recognised.

Relapse of symptoms

This indicates a recurrence of previous symptoms, the enhancement of existing ones, or the development of new ones after a period of relative quiescence, provided that they persist for more than 3 days. A relapse is described as acute when the advance of previous symptoms is abrupt, so that previous disability or distress is significantly increased within 24 hours, or the development of new symptoms leads to functional disability or distress within this time. When the symptoms that develop or recur persist for less than 3 days, the episode is described as a transient exacerbation rather than a relapse.

Partial or complete remission

This describes a partial improvement or complete clearing of symptoms for more than 3 days, provided that these symptoms had themselves been present for at least this period of time. When a regression of symptoms occurs but persists for less than 3 days, it is described as a transient improvement.

Progressive course

This refers to the advance in severity of existing symptoms or the development of new ones with time. Such a course is described as steadily progressive when it is not associated with more than one acute relapse, and as episodic if two or more acute relapses occur during it.

Clinical onset and course

Although symptoms commenced insidiously in the great majority of cases, they did develop acutely in some instances. A more precise assessment of the relative frequency of these two modes of onset could not be made because in a number of cases pain was the first symptom of the angioma and preceded other symptoms by many years, thereby making it difficult to define the manner of onset with any certainty. Accordingly, it seemed more useful to characterise the onset and development of those symptoms with which patients eventually presented. These commenced acutely in 12 patients and developed more gradually in the remaining 48, one of whom, however, gave a past history of recurrent subarachnoid haemorrhage. They subsequently continued to advance in severity up to the time of diagnosis in all but 7 patients, each of whom presented with disability of acute onset.

Sargent (1925) drew attention to the remarkable variability of symptoms which sometimes occurs over short periods of time, as in one of his own cases in which symptoms varied from hour to hour. In several patients in the present series, there was some fluctuation in the severity of symptoms over short intervals (i.e. less than 72 hours), either in relation to specific factors such as exercise or posture as described in Chapter 8, or without obvious cause, but this fluctuation occurred against a background of steadily increasing disability.

PROGRESSIVE COURSE

Symptoms progressed steadily from their onset up to the time of diagnosis in 53 cases, but in 5 this course was interrupted by an acute relapse. Another 6 of these patients recalled a previous brief neurological disturbance other than pain, which in some had occurred a number of years before the onset and advance of symptoms with which they eventually presented; in another patient, already referred to above, there was a history of recurrent subarachnoid haemorrhage in the 17 years before he developed the progressive limb weakness with which he presented.

Wyburn-Mason (1943) considered that a discontinuity of symptoms was one of the cardinal features of the history in patients with a spinal angioma, progression occurring characteristically—but not always—by a series of 'apoplectiform stages' with, at least initially, intervening periods of remission. This is consistent with the clinical experience of several other authors, including Djindjian, Hurth and Houdart (1970) who emphasised that the essential feature common to these episodes was their involvement of the same level of the spinal cord. Analysis of these and earlier reports reveals that relapses may occur at any time after the initial symptoms, and that their character and severity are not influenced by that of earlier episodes although they relate to the same level of the cord.

Apart from the cases mentioned above, a discontinuity of symptoms was not conspicuous in the present series of cases except with respect to pain, which was often intermittent. Moreover, an episodic progression of symptoms did not really occur in any patient, although several recognised milestones during their downhill course, when they first appreciated that their functional capacity had become more restricted. This accords with the experience of Arseni and Samitca (1959) who found that a slow steady deterioration occurred in all but 2 of their 18 patients, and with that of Newman (1959) who reported that the clinical course in his 19 patients was one of steadily progressive deterioration, with a major remission occurring in only one instance.

This apparent disagreement may relate in part to differences in terminology and to the difficulties inherent in interpreting individual case histories. Nevertheless, it seems reasonable to conclude that progression of symptoms may occur either steadily or episodically, with or without intervening periods of remission.

NON-PROGRESSIVE COURSE

In 7 patients presenting symptoms were acute in onset but had not advanced further by the time of diagnosis. The subsequent course in these patients is therefore of particular interest. Two presented with a paraparesis, but each recovered sufficiently well to lead a completely unrestricted life for the 5 and 8 years that they have since remained under medical supervision. A third patient presented with a sensory and sphincter disturbance which similarly remitted spontaneously, and she has remained well over the subsequent 17 years. The remaining 4 patients have each remained moderately or severely disabled from a paraparesis of acute onset, but no further developments have occurred over follow-up periods of 16, 13, 8 and 5 years respectively.

The eventual outcome in these patients cannot be viewed with complacency, however, for further symptoms may yet develop. As indicated above, several patients in this series recalled a previous neurological incident from which they recovered completely, only to develop further symptoms at a later date. One of these patients, described in detail in the Appendix (p. 148), made a complete recovery from a paraparesis of acute onset and remained well for 28 years before developing the symptoms with which he eventually presented. The experience of such authors as Wyburn-Mason (1943) and Djindjian, Hurth and Houdart (1970) similarly suggests that the risks of an acute relapse remain, even though no developments have yet occurred.

Prognosis

It is important to obtain some insight into the rate and extent of progression of symptoms, and to the severity of

incapacity which results in untreated cases, because
these aspects of the natural history are of direct relevance
to the management of patients with a spinal angioma.
It is difficult, however, to compare satisfactorily the
severity of symptoms such as paraesthesiae in different
patients or in individual patients at different times,
because their subjective nature precludes a uniform
manner of assessment. This aspect was therefore neglected, and progression was assessed by reference only to
the degree of disability. For this purpose direct enquiry
about disability was made to patients or their general
practitioners, unless they had continued to attend hospital
for regular follow-up after the diagnosis was established.
Some patients had undergone exploratory or decompressive laminectomy but, as indicated in Chapter 12, it is
generally accepted that these procedures confer no
therapeutic benefit; these patients were therefore considered as untreated for the purpose of this study.
When patients had undergone corrective procedures
such as excision of the malformation or ligation of its
feeding arteries, however, the outcome was studied only
to the time of operation. The mean duration of the history
for the whole series was 8 years.

GAIT

In patients with a progressive history the mean interval
between the first symptom of any sort and the most severe
permanent disorder of gait which they developed was 5·7
years, but in some instances vague, intermittent pain
had preceded other symptoms by several years. In the
following discussion, therefore, progression of disability
has been related to the onset of leg weakness or disturbed
gait, whichever was earlier, since this was recalled more
definitely and was attributable solely to the angioma
with more justification.

The rate of progression varied considerably, but in
about half of the cases it was so rapid that individual
disability had reached its maximum within one year,
showing little change thereafter in untreated patients.

The extent of progression also showed considerable
individual differences, but 33 of the 60 patients eventually
became so permanently disabled that they either required
2 sticks or crutches for walking, or were unable to walk
at all. The time course over which this severe degree
of disability developed is indicated in Table 9.1. It is
likely that further progression would have occurred in
some of the remaining 27 patients with milder disability

Table 9.1. Development
of severe disturbance of
gait in 33 patients.

| | *Number of patients* | |
	Unable to walk without 2 sticks or crutches	Unable to walk at all. Confined to bed or chair
Time from onset of leg weakness or gait disturbance		
0–6 months	3	7
6–12 months	1	4
1–2 years		3
2–3 years	3	7
3–4 years		1
4–5 years		2
5+ years	1	1
Total number of patients	8	25

Note The above data relate to the greatest disability which developed in each case, so that no patient has been counted more than once.

if the follow-up period had been longer or they had not been operated upon.

Progression may thus occur with great rapidity or more slowly, and may lead either to severe incapacity or to less conspicuous disability such as a reduced exercise tolerance, with little change occurring thereafter. The following case history illustrates the rapidity with which severe disability may sometimes develop.

A housewife, aged 59 years, gave a 6 month history of urgency and frequency of micturition, together with progressive difficulty in walking, and a 2 month history of paraesthesiae in both legs. The gait disturbance had advanced steadily and become so severe that she was confined to bed for the 2 weeks prior to her admission to the National Hospital (83069). Examination revealed complete paralysis of both legs with absent tendon reflexes and bilateral extensor plantar responses, gross postural loss in the legs, and impaired appreciation of vibration below the costal margin. Myelography and exploratory laminectomy revealed the presence of a lower thoracic angioma which was left undisturbed. She died 3 months later.

A contrast is provided by the next case, in which severe disability developed much more slowly.

A grocer, aged 44 years, gave a 15 month history of slowly progressive weakness which commenced quite suddenly and immediately caused him to drag his legs while walking. It was accompanied by some difficulty in micturition and defaecation, and was followed after a few months by impotence and then by gradually increasing numbness of the legs. He was admitted to Atkinson Morley's Hospital (A 19168) where examination revealed a mild spastic paraparesis and slight hypalgesia in the legs, but myelography showed no definite abnormality and he was discharged. He was readmitted after 2½ years because his legs had become steadily weaker although he was still able to get about with a stick, and he had developed occasional urinary incontinence due to impaired sensation of bladder fullness. Examination confirmed that his motor deficit had increased, and all modalities of sensation were impaired bilaterally below the 12th thoracic dermatome. Myelography on this occasion showed the typical appearance of a lower thoracic angioma which was considered inoperable, and he returned home. His condition continued to deteriorate, but he was still able to get about with a stick 2 years later, although with much more difficulty and for shorter distances than previously. Over the following 2–3 years, however, his disability increased further, and eventually he became confined to a wheel-chair and required a permanent in-dwelling catheter. He died 7 years later, 16 years after the onset of his symptoms, and autopsy confirmed the presence of an angioma. Finally, the next case illustrates the insidious development of mild disability, with little change occurring thereafter.

A 64-year old company director gave a 3 year history of mild weakness and numbness in the left leg, as a result of which he had taken to walking with a stick for support. His symptoms, which developed insidiously, were aggravated by standing still for longer than 10 minutes, or by walking for 400 yards, and were relieved by resting for 2 minutes. On admission to the National Hospital (73856), examination revealed weakness of the left hip flexor muscles, an absent left ankle jerk and a depressed right one, but no other signs. Myelography demonstrated a lumbar angioma which was confirmed by laminectomy, but the malformation was not disturbed. There has been no change in the nature or severity of his symptoms over the subsequent 17 years.

The rate of progression may change during the course of the disorder. Symptoms which have slowly advanced in severity over many years may begin to progress more rapidly so that severe disability results over a few weeks, as in the following case.

A retired millwright, aged 73 years, gave a 4 year history of weakness, numbness and pain in the legs. His symptoms commenced insidiously, gradually advancing in severity to restrict his exercise tolerance, but he nevertheless remained able to get about. Nine weeks prior to admission, however, the weakness gradually became more severe until eventually he was able to move only his toes, his sensory symptoms became more troublesome, and he developed a sphincter disturbance which culminated in urinary retention and faecal incontinence. He was admitted to Maida Vale Hospital (52009) where examination revealed an almost complete flaccid paraplegia, with gross wasting of all muscle groups in the legs, complete analgesia up to the 1st right and 2nd left lumbar dermatomes, impaired joint position sense to the knees, and loss of vibration appreciation below the costal margin. Myelography revealed the typical appearances of a spinal angioma in the lower thoracic region.

The rate at which a disturbance of gait developed was studied further by determining in each case the time that elapsed from its onset, or the onset of leg weakness, before persisting disability was at its greatest. Four of the 60 patients were excluded from this part of the study, 2 because they had never had any leg weakness or difficulty with walking, and 2 others because they had experienced a disturbance of gait for only a very brief period before operation. The 6 patients, described earlier, who presented with a paraparesis that commenced acutely but failed to progress, were included, however, because they subsequently remained with some disturbance of gait.

Within 6 months of its onset, at least 10 of these 56 patients were unable to walk at all, or required 2 sticks or crutches to get about, and the number known to be so disabled had risen to 28 (50 per cent) in less than 3 years (Table 9.2). Disability did not become as severe as this in the remaining 28 cases, but it was sufficient nevertheless to interfere with daily activity in most; within a period of up to 3 years, 12 had developed a reduced exercise tolerance, 11 needed the support of a stick to walk, and only 5 had a milder degree of incapacity. Moreover, the history was of relatively short duration in 4 of these 28 patients, and it is likely that further progression would have occurred if they had not been operated upon. These observations are consistent with the experience of Newman (1959) who found that 11 of his 19 patients (58 per cent) were completely unable to walk within periods ranging from 6 months to 4 years after they had first noticed leg weakness.

Table 9.2. Severity of gait disturbance at various intervals after its onset.

	Number of patients Interval from onset		
	Up to 6 months	Up to 3 years	Unlimited*
Total number of patients for whom information was available	52	56	56
Greatest disability:			
leg weakness, abnormal stance or gait, without restriction of exercise tolerance	29 (56%)	5 (9%)	2 (4%)
restricted exercise tolerance	11 (21%)	12 (21%)	9 (16%)
needing 1 stick or some support to walk	2 (4%)	11 (20%)	12 (21%)
unable to walk without 2 sticks or crutches	3 (6%)	7 (13%)	8 (14%)
unable to walk at all; confined to bed or chair	7 (13%)	21 (37%)	25 (45%)

* Duration of history until treatment, loss to follow-up or time of the study.

The implications of these observations are clear. The great majority of patients with a spinal angioma can expect their daily activities and capabilities to become increasingly restricted, often to a considerable extent and over a relatively short period of time, if the malformation is left untreated after leg weakness or a disturbance of gait has first become noticeable.

DISTURBANCES OF MICTURITION AND DEFAECATION

These occurred at any time in relation to the onset and progression of somatic symptoms, and although they were often particularly severe in patients with a marked disturbance of gait, they nevertheless constituted the major disability in some cases.

A disturbance of micturition developed in 56 of the 60 patients in this series, but in 18 it remained mild, consisting solely of hesitancy, urgency and/or frequency. Of the remainder, 12 had occasional urinary incontinence or retention, and 26 became totally incontinent or developed persistent retention; these more incapacitating symptoms arose *de novo* in approximately half of these 38 patients, while in the remainder they followed milder symptoms which had advanced in severity with time. For example, 12 of the 26 patients with total incontinence or persistent retention had not had any previous disturbance of micturition, and in 10 of the remaining 14 patients mild symptoms were followed by this degree of incapacity within 2 years of their onset.

A disturbance of defaecation developed in 42 patients, but in 19 this consisted solely of mild constipation. In 15 patients there was occasional faecal incontinence or intractable constipation of such severity that several had resorted to attempts at removing faeces manually, In another 8 patients there was complete faecal incontinence, and this arose *de novo* in 5 cases.

Clearly, the risk of developing a severe disturbance of micturition and/or defaecation is not inconsiderable in patients with a spinal angioma; such a disturbance may develop at any time, and need not be preceded by milder, warning symptoms. Thus, almost half of the patients in this series became either totally incontinent of urine or developed persistent retention, and in about half of these patients there was no prior warning that the control of micturition was disturbed in any way. The great majority of these patients had caudally situated angiomas, however, and these conclusions do not necessarily apply to patients with a malformation in the cervical region.

SUBARACHNOID HAEMORRHAGE

This occurred in 6 patients, in 3 of whom it was the first symptom of the angioma, and was the terminal event in one case. It was recurrent in only one patient, who experienced six haemorrhages over 17 years from a cervical angioma—and was twice investigated elsewhere by carotid and vertebral angiography—before he developed signs of an intramedullary disturbance of cord function. Spinal subarachnoid haemorrhage has been discussed in detail in Chapter 7, and further comment here is therefore unnecessary.

Prognostic guides

An attempt was made to identify factors that might provide a guide to prognosis at an early stage in the natural history of the disorder, and thus facilitate the early recognition of patients destined to develop severe incapacity.

AGE AND SEX

Of the 12 women in this series, 9 developed a disturbance of gait or weakness in the legs which remained troublesome. Four of these 9 patients were unable to walk at all within 6 months, and 6 were incapacitated to this extent in less than 3 years. In contrast, 47 of the 48 male patients developed a gait disorder, but only 3 were chair-bound within 6 months, and 15 within 3 years. This suggests that once leg weakness or a disturbance of gait has begun to develop, female patients fare less well than males, but no firm conclusions can be drawn because of the small numbers involved.

There were only 11 patients aged 40 years or less at the time of diagnosis, but of the 7 who developed a permanent disturbance of gait, 4 were chair-bound within 3 years. This is a much higher incidence than in the series as a whole, but there was an equal sex distribution among these younger patients in contrast to the male preponderance among older ones, and this may have influenced the outcome. In any event, the small numbers again involved do not permit any general conclusions to be reached.

It was not possible to reach a more definite conclusion about these points by studying the literature because of the paucity of clinical details provided in many cases.

FLUCTUATION OF SYMPTOMS

In several patients symptoms fluctuated in intensity over short periods of time, and this occurred either spontaneously or, more commonly, in relation to exercise or certain postures. Clinical impression suggested that cord function was precarious in many of these patients, but in no case did such a fluctuation of symptoms presage an acute relapse or any obvious change in the rate of progression.

LOCATION OF ANGIOMA

In the great majority of patients in this series, the angioma was located in the thoracic or lumbar region, and the number of patients with a cervical angioma was too small to permit any conclusions to be reached concerning the manner in which the level of the malformation influenced the eventual outcome. It will be recalled from Chapter 5, though, that angiomas in the cervical and upper thoracic region are usually diagnosed at a much earlier age than more caudal lesions; this suggests that they lead to the earlier development of symptoms which warrant investigation, and by inference, therefore, to earlier—but not necessarily to greater—disability. There is also a higher incidence of subarachnoid haemorrhage from angiomas in this region, but this in itself is probably not the usual cause for their earlier diagnosis because the spinal source of the haemorrhage is very often unrecognised until symptoms and signs of cord dysfunction develop, as discussed in Chapter 7.

ANGIOGRAPHY

Only 12 of the 60 patients studied were investigated by selective angiography and it was not possible to correlate the radiographic features of the malformation with the natural history and outcome in these cases.

The presence of several feeding arteries, the rapid opacification of draining veins, and the relatively fast clearance of contrast medium suggests that an angioma contains a shunt of large volume. These angiographic features are frequently found in patients with a cervical or upper thoracic angioma, who usually develop symptoms—and presumably some degree of disability—at a relatively early age, and also in children or young adults irrespective of the location of the angioma. Moreover, when subarachnoid haemorrhage occurs, it is usually from an angioma with a shunt of large volume. The angiographic features may therefore be of some practical value when the benefits of surgical treatment are being considered in patients with inconspicuous symptoms and no disability, by indicating which patients are more liable to subarachnoid haemorrhage or the early development of other neurological symptoms.

Mortality

Twenty of the 60 patients studied are known to have died, but in 7 the cause of death could not be determined from the available records, and in another 3 cases it was unrelated to the angioma. Of the remaining 10 patients, one died from a spinal subarachnoid haemorrhage and 9 from one of the complications of chronic paraplegia. The risks of premature death have been much reduced by recent advances in the care of paraplegic patients, and further comment is therefore unnecessary here.

Summary

1 The natural history of spinal angiomas has been studied by reference to the medical records of 60 cases, and the findings are contrasted with those of earlier

authors. It is concluded that symptoms may develop abruptly or insidiously, and may fluctuate in intensity over short intervals. They usually advance in severity with time, but this progression may occur steadily or episodically, with or without intervening periods of remission. In some cases there may be no progression for many years, but the risk remains that disability will eventually develop, either acutely or more gradually.

2 A permanent disturbance of gait occurred in 56 of the patients studied. The rate at which this progressed from its onset varied considerably, but in about half of these cases it had reached its maximum within one year. The degree of disability was such that 33 patients eventually became unable to walk at all, or needed 2 sticks or crutches to do so; this developed in 10 patients within 6 months, and in 28 within 3 years of its onset. In the remaining 23 patients, the disability that developed was usually sufficient to interfere with normal daily activities. This suggests that once leg weakness or a disturbance of gait has become noticeable, the daily activities and capabilities of patients with a spinal angioma will usually become increasingly restricted—often very rapidly and to a severe degree—unless the underlying lesion is treated.

3 Disturbances of micturition and defaecation were common, were sometimes severely incapacitating from their onset, and developed at any time in relation to the onset and progression of somatic symptoms.

4 Severe incapacity occurred more commonly in female or young patients, but the numbers involved were too small to permit any general conclusions to be reached. No other clinical guides to prognosis could be recognised from the present case material. The previously published data indicate, however, that cervical angiomas become symptomatic earlier than more caudal lesions, thereby suggesting that they lead to disablement at an earlier age. The angiographic feature of the malformations may also be of prognostic significance in indicating those which are likely to lead to subarachnoid haemorrhage or the early development of other neurological symptoms.

Chapter 10
Pathology of spinal angiomas

The pathological features of spinal angiomas, and the disturbances to which they lead in the structure and function of the spinal cord may now be considered in detail and related to the clinical features described in the previous two chapters. As indicated in Chapter 1, telangiectases and cavernous angiomas will not be discussed, for the only type of hamartoma under consideration consists of an abnormal arteriovenous communication which permits arterial blood to enter the venous system without passing through a capillary network. In some of these angiomas an artery opens directly into a vein, but in the majority a cluster of dilated vessels, which are difficult to classify, is interposed between normal arteries and veins.

In about 70 per cent of cases the shunt is situated at or below the level of the 9th thoracic segment of the cord. It is usually extramedullary, but it is difficult to make an accurate assessment of the proportion of cases in which it is located within the cord. Large, abnormal vessels may be seen at angiography to penetrate the cord, and surgical exploration sometimes reveals conspicuous connections between vessels on the cord's surface and those within it, but this does not necessarily imply that the shunt is intramedullary, for such vessels may be draining or feeding a purely extramedullary one; the presence of local swelling of the cord makes it more likely, however, that part of the angioma is intramedullary. These abnormal vessels must not be confused with the finer ones which are usually found connecting the cord with the angiomatous extramedullary vessels at operation, for the latter probably represent the channels through which the cord normally drains to veins in the pia. Post-mortem examination sometimes reveals an angioma situated within the cord, but pathological studies have been too few to permit any assessment of the frequency with which this occurs. Moreover, it has not always been appreciated that extensive pathological changes may be present within the cord even though the angioma is entirely extramedullary.

The most reliable data on this point are probably that of Djindjian, Houdart and Hurth (1969) relating to 50 cases studied angiographically, 29 of which were subsequently operated upon. These authors found that in only 8 per cent of their 50 cases was the lesion mainly or completely intramedullary, although in a number of other cases abnormal vessels were said to penetrate the cord, and in a more recent review of his experience Djindjian (1972) indicated that 80 per cent of angiomas were situated posterior to the cord and could be excised completely.

Pathological anatomy

The present account is based in part on those of Wyburn-Mason (1943), Brion, Netsky and Zimmerman (1952), and Antoni (1962), and in part on the pathological findings in 5 cases which came to autopsy, and 16 cases in which the malformation was excised at the National Hospitals for Nervous Diseases.

EXTRAMEDULLARY ANGIOMAS

Macroscopic appearance

When the dura is opened at autopsy, a mass of distended, tortuous vessels is usually seen within the leptomeninges and overlying the spinal cord (Figure 10.1), but in some cases only a single coiled vessel is present, particularly in the thoraco-lumbar region. These vessels may be localised to a few segments or extend the whole length of the cord, and may penetrate the cord or run between and with the nerve roots. They are usually situated posteriorly but in some instances, particularly in the cervical and upper thoracic regions, are more conspicuous anteriorly. They may be embedded in the subjacent cord and appear to have compressed it, but this is rare.

It is often difficult to decide whether a particular vessel is arterial or venous in character, and it is not usually possible to recognise the actual site of the abnormal fistulous communication between the arterial and venous systems except by injection techniques. In some instances, however, an artery can be seen to run to this collection of vessels or directly into a vein, as in a case reported by Antoni (1962) in which a branch of the anterior spinal artery opened directly into an enormous venous varix in the upper thoracic region. Blood from the angioma drains usually to prominent and distended veins on the posterior and lateral surfaces of the cord and thence to the medullary veins accompanying the nerve roots, but in some cases it drains directly to veins situated anteriorly.

The cord itself may be swollen due to haemorrhage, oedema or to an intramedullary component of the malformation, or shrunken due to ischaemic necrosis, and there may be leptomeningeal thickening, discolouration or adhesions. On sectioning it, areas of haemorrhage

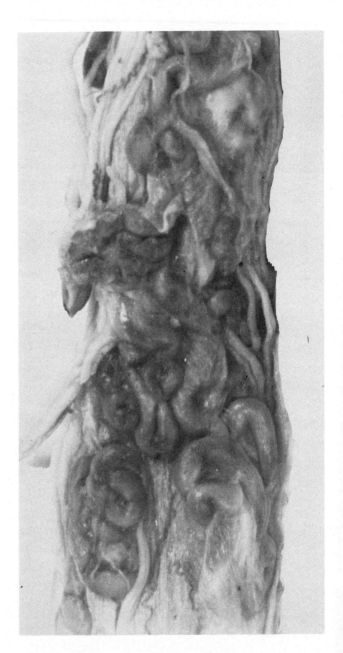

Figure 10.1. Enlarged, tortuous vessels on the posterior surface of the thoracic cord.

or infarction, or a localised collection of abnormal vessels may immediately be evident, but in other instances no gross abnormality is seen.

Microscopic appearances

The vessels on the surface of the cord are usually deformed and atypical, with hypertrophied walls of irregular thickness (Figure 10.2), and some may be occluded by

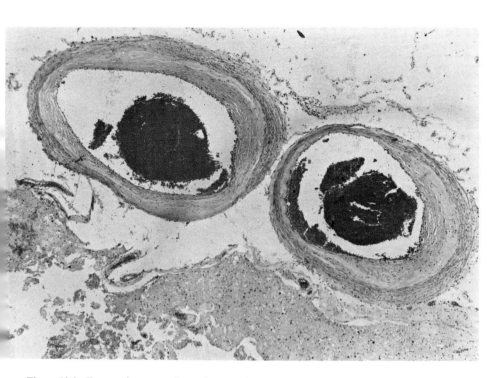

Figure 10.2. Two angiomatous vessels, with hypertrophied walls of irregular thickness, in the leptomeninges (haematoxylin and eosin; × 24).

thrombus. They may consist solely of collagenous connective tissue lined by a single layer of endothelium, but the presence of smooth muscle and elastic tissue sometimes gives them an arterial structure. In vessels that are obviously arterial, the internal elastic lamina may be reduplicated, frayed or disrupted, and the muscle layer is often irregular in thickness and sometimes contains areas of calcification. Even when the fistulous portion of the malformation is examined, the actual point of transition from artery to vein can rarely be appreciated.

The abnormalities found within the cord are illustrated in Figures 10.3–10.6. The most consistent is the presence of numerous veins, venules, and capillary-sized vessels with thickened, hyalinised walls which are sometimes infiltrated with round cells, and these vessels may be arranged in clusters or clumps. This apparent proliferation of vessels is often found over a considerable length of the cord, but in the transverse axis it is sometimes particularly prominent in posterior and lateral regions (Brion, Netsky and Zimmerman, 1952; Aminoff, Barnard and Logue, 1974) so that the antero-medial segment appears to be relatively spared, unless the angioma itself is situated anteriorly. Degeneration of nerve cell bodies and axons, and demyelination of fibre tracts occur to a variable extent, and glial proliferation is

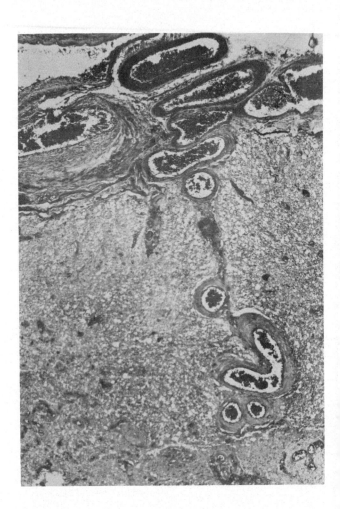

Figure 10.3. A group of abnormal vessels on the surface of the cord. Intramedullary vessels are dilated (Elastic—van Gieson; ×82).

sometimes extensive. Thrombotic occlusion of intramedullary vessels of all types and sizes is a conspicuous feature in some cases, but is completely absent in others. Cystic infarction, or evidence of old or recent haemorrhage may be found, and in advanced stages the normal structure of the cord is completely lost. It should be emphasised that the distribution of these pathological changes does not correspond to the territory supplied by any of the named spinal arteries.

INTRAMEDULLARY ANGIOMAS

Although the precise location of the abnormal shunt cannot usually be determined without angiography or post-mortem injection procedures, in some cases the presence within the cord of a localised collection of sinusoidal vascular channels, and enlarged arteries and veins of abnormal structure, separated by neural par-

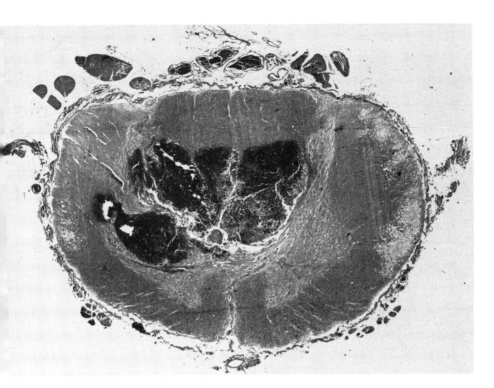

Figure 10.4. Transverse section of cervical cord. There is a large, central, intramedullary haemorrhage. Tract degeneration is seen in the lateral columns (Luxol fast blue, haematoxylin and eosin, × 11).

enchyma, suggests that it is intramedullary (Figure 10.7). In such cases the pathological findings are otherwise similar to those described above, except that the vessels on the surface of the cord are usually less conspicuous than in patients with an extramedullary angioma, and sometimes look relatively normal.

Pathophysiology

The manner in which the underlying fistula leads to a disturbance of function in the spinal cord is uncertain, and will be discussed in this section. Further experience may modify the pathophysiological concept which is speculatively advanced, but this does not detract from any value that it may have in aiding the formulation of experimental studies to increase knowledge about these lesions.

DIMINISHED INTRAMEDULLARY ARTERIOVENOUS PRESSURE GRADIENT

The majority of spinal angiomas are situated posteriorly and drain directly or indirectly to pial veins on the posterior and lateral surfaces of the cord. As shown in Figure 10.8, the anomalous arteriovenous shunt must lead to

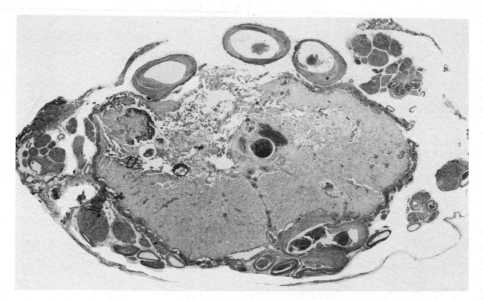

Figure 10.5. Transverse section of the 8th thoracic segment of the cord. Large, abnormal vessels are present in the leptomeninges, and the posterior columns of the cord are infarcted. The cord tissue in the region of the anterior median fissure is relatively well preserved (phosphotungstic acid haematoxylin; × 11).

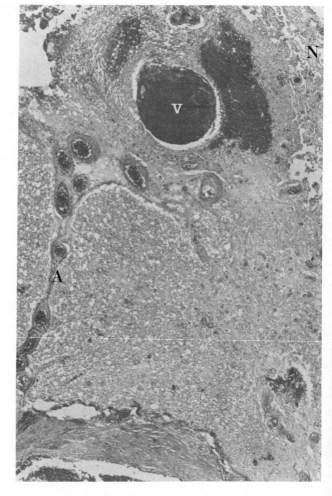

Figure 10.6. Part of transverse section of thoracic cord. Thrombosis of an intramedullary vessel (V) with adjacent haemorrhage and necrosis (N) is seen. The cord tissue adjacent to the anterior median fissure (A) is preserved (phosphotungistic acid haematoxylin; × 22).

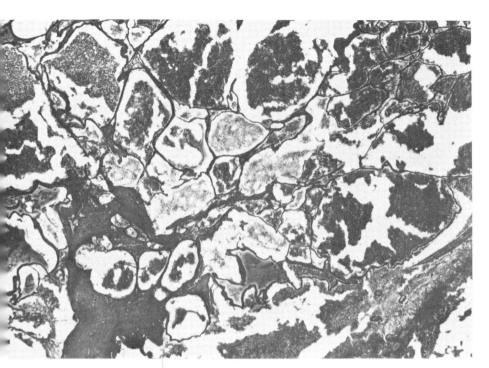

Figure 10.7. Part of an intramedullary angioma. A reticulin framework separates large blood spaces (reticulin; × 46).

an increased pressure in these veins and, since they form part of an intercommunicating plexus that also drains the intramedullary circulation, to an associated rise in intramedullary venous pressure. The consequent reduction in the intramedullary arteriovenous pressure gradient will presumably lead to a reduced intramedullary blood flow, and thus to ischaemia of the spinal cord (Aminoff, Barnard and Logue, 1974).

The clinical features of spinal angiomas are fully consistent with this hypothesis, for they indicate that there is a disturbance of function in the cord which extends beyond the territory of any of the named spinal arteries but is similar in distribution to the pattern of intramedullary venous drainage. Moreover, the rapid fluctuations in the severity of symptoms which may occur over short intervals of time are readily explicable in terms of a disturbance of flow.

The nature and distribution of the pathological changes described above also accord well with this hypothesis. It is generally accepted that neuronal degeneration, axonal demyelination, and an apparent proliferation of small vessels occur in ischaemic lesions of the central nervous system, and the presence of tissue necrosis and cystic infarction confirms that the cord is sometimes severely ischaemic. Hyaline thickening of vessel walls may also be due to ischaemia, or to an increased intraluminal pressure. As indicated above, intravascular thrombosis is a conspicuous finding at autopsy in some, but not other cases, and this presumably relates to slowing of the circulation, and perhaps also to structural changes in vessel walls.

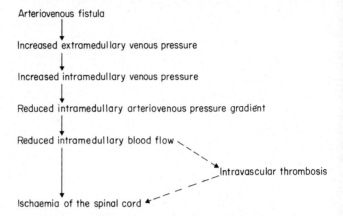

Figure 10.8. Diagrammatic representation of the proposed sequence of changes leading to cord ischaemia in patients with a spinal angioma.

As discussed in Chapter 2, the venous drainage of the antero-medial segment of the cord is initially distinct from that of the remainder; the former drains to the anterior median spinal vein, while the rest of the cord drains by radial veins to the intercommunicating plexus of coronal veins situated posteriorly and laterally in the pia. Accordingly, the antero-medial part of the cord (medial cell columns of the anterior horns and white matter of the anterior funiculi) will often be less severely affected than the remainder if the pathological changes described earlier are indeed due to venous back pressure (cf. Gillilan, 1970), although it will certainly be involved to some extent because of the anastomoses which exist between the extrinsic spinal cord veins. Detailed histological examination in one case confirmed that there was relative sparing in this region (Aminoff, Barnard and Logue, 1974), but it was not possible to determine whether this was the rule by studying the previously published case reports, because of the paucity of detail usually provided.

OTHER CONCEPTS

The symptoms of patients with a spinal angioma have been attributed to ischaemia of the cord occurring for other reasons, or to cord compression, and these concepts merit careful consideration.

Thrombosis

Symptoms have been related to intravascular thrombosis (Wyburn-Mason, 1943), but the rapid fluctuations in their severity which sometimes occur are difficult to account for on this basis alone, and in some cases (Brion, Netsky and Zimmerman, 1952; Aminoff, Barnard and Logue, 1974) thrombotic lesions are either absent or inconspicuous at post-mortem examination. In 1926 Foix and Alajouanine described 2 cases of subacute necrotic myelitis in which hypertrophied, tortuous pial vessels were associated with intramedullary changes of the type described above, and specifically commented on the lack of thrombotic lesions in their pathological material. It is therefore of interest that this condition is now usually attributed to the presence of an underlying angioma (Wyburn-Mason, 1943; Antoni, 1962; Wirth, Post, Di Chiro, Doppman and Ommaya, 1970).

These observations make it unlikely that thrombosis is the prime cause of cord ischaemia, although it doubtless enhances any pre-existing ischaemia when it does occur.

Steal

It has been suggested that blood is preferentially diverted to the angioma from the normal spinal circulation as a 'steal' phenomenon, thereby leading to ischaemia of the cord (Shephard, 1963; Krayenbühl, Yaşargil and McClintock, 1969; Chatterjee and Roy, 1968; Djindjian, Hurth and Houdart, 1970), but several factors suggest that this is not the usual cause of symptoms.

Most spinal angiomas are situated posteriorly, but steal from the posterior spinal circulation would hardly account for the symptoms and signs to which they usually lead, nor for the widely distributed changes found at autopsy; moreover, the posterior spinal arteries—in contrast to the anterior—are well supplied by a number of segmental feeding vessels in each of the three longitudinal arterial territories of the cord, and steal from one of these would therefore be unlikely to lead to cord ischaemia. Steal could perhaps occur if the anterior spinal artery itself supplied the angioma, but this is uncommon (Doppman, Di Chiro and Ommaya, 1969; Logue, Aminoff and Kendall, 1974) except in the cervical region (Djindjian, Hurth and Houdart, 1970). It is similarly uncommon for the artery feeding the angioma to arise as a branch of one supplying the anterior spinal, or for these two arteries to arise from the same segmental stem, except in the cervical region, so that steal will not normally occur by this route. It could occur through collateral vessels if these arteries arose from adjacent segmental vessels, but the clinical features of patients with a spinal angioma are not consistent with the anterior spinal artery syndrome, and the pathological findings at autopsy do not correspond in their distribution with the territory supplied by this artery.

It is conceivable that steal occurs through vessels connecting the intramedullary circulation with that in the angioma, but such interconnections are inconspicuous at operation in many cases. Moreover, if steal did occur by this route, ligation of the main segmental feeders of the angioma might augment it due to a reduction in pressure in the angioma, whereas therapeutic benefit usually follows this procedure (Ommaya, Di Chiro and Doppman, 1969). Although ligation of feeding vessels might reduce steal due to suction produced in a manner analogous to the operation of a laboratory filter-pump (in which water flowing rapidly through a tube produces suction in a connected side-tube), the relatively slow flow through many caudally situated angiomas makes it improbable that significant steal would occur by this means even if the two circulations were interconnected.

It seems reasonable to conclude that although steal may occur in some instances, it is unlikely to be the prime cause of symptoms in patients with a spinal angioma.

Cord compression

Some authors (Shephard, 1963; Doppman, Di Chiro and Ommaya, 1969) have suggested that the spinal cord is compressed by enlarged pial vessels, and such a concept is clearly implicit in the previous surgical practice of treating spinal angiomas by decompressive procedures. However, manometric or myelographic evidence of obstruction in the subarachnoid space is uncommon, the usual finding at operation is of coiled vessels which occupy only part of the subarachnoid space and are not even in contact with the inelastic dura, and there is often little evidence of compression when the cord is examined at autopsy. It is hardly surprising therefore that decompression was usually ineffective in arresting the steady advance of symptoms in patients with these malformations.

Clinicopathological correlations

Some of the clinical aspects which were discussed in earlier chapters are tentatively interpreted below in terms of the pathological features and pathophysiological concept just described, but many of these correlations must be regarded as no more than working hypotheses which await adequate verification. Furthermore, it is not clear why many patients remain asymptomatic until middle age or even longer, although this may reflect age-related changes in blood flow to the cord or angioma, or in the regional requirements of blood by the cord.

ACUTE ONSET OR EXACERBATION OF SYMPTOMS

It seems probable that this is sometimes due to episodes of intramedullary haemorrhage, which can certainly occur without clinical evidence of associated bleeding into the subarachnoid space and may thus pass unrecognised until the cord is examined at autopsy. It may also result from the thrombotic occlusion of a major extramedullary vessel, as in the case reported by Rand (1927) which is summarised on p. 61; surgical exploration soon after the acute onset of a paraparesis in a patient seen recently at the National Hospital similarly revealed that a large extramedullary vessel was occluded by fresh thrombus. Thrombosis of major intramedullary vessels can presumably also lead to the abrupt advance of symptoms, but this is more difficult to corroborate.

STEADY PROGRESSION OF SYMPTOMS

This relates to increasing cord ischaemia due to the reduced intramedullary blood flow, aggravated in some cases by the thrombotic occlusion of increasing numbers of small intramedullary vessels. The rapid, spontaneous fluctuation in the severity of symptoms which occurs in some patients probably reflects the slight variations which constantly occur in local blood flow or requirements. When the malformation is mainly intramedullary, symptoms may also arise by displacement of adjacent structures. Symptoms sometimes have a radicular distribution, presumably because there is ischaemia of a nerve root or because the root is compressed by enlarged vessels, particularly within the confines of the intervertebral foramen.

Trauma

Trauma can induce thrombosis, haemorrhage, or alterations of regional blood flow, and any one of these factors may underlie the temporal relationship that symptoms sometimes have to injury.

Exercise

Ischaemia due to a reduced intramedullary blood flow is enhanced at times of increased requirements such as during exercise. This occurs either because intrinsic autoregulatory mechanisms are unable to compensate further to meet these additional needs in full, or because they have themselves failed due to the underlying ischaemic process.

Posture

The size and configuration of the spinal canal and intervertebral foramina vary with posture (Jellinger and Neumayer, 1972), and biomechanical factors may thus explain the aggravation of symptoms by posture. In particular, compression of draining veins, especially those accompanying the nerve roots, will increase venous back pressure, so that the intramedullary arteriovenous pressure gradient is reduced still further and cord ischaemia is transiently increased.

Pregnancy

Pressure by the enlarged uterus on the pelvic and abdominal veins may aggravate symptoms by impeding venous return to the heart and thereby reducing further the intramedullary arteriovenous pressure gradient in patients with a caudally situated angioma. In addition, haemodilution and anaemia will enhance any pre-existing cord ischaemia. Newman (1958) has suggested that hormonal changes also aggravate symptoms, but little direct evidence is available on this point.

Increase in body temperature

Symptoms are sometimes aggravated by a febrile illness or by hot baths, and this probably relates to a reversible conduction block induced in demyelinated fibres by the rise in body temperature, such as occurs in experimentally demyelinated root fibres in the rat (Rasminsky, 1973).

Valsalva's manoeuvre

A forced expiration against a closed glottis increases the intrathoracic pressure and thus impedes the venous return to the heart. This leads to an increase in pressure in veins draining the cord and angioma, and accordingly to a further reduction in intramedullary blood flow. Valsalva's manoeuvre is performed when straining at stool, and often when holding the breath, and presumably accounts for the occasional exacerbation of symptoms which occurs in patients at these times. This manoeuvre may also be of practical value in enabling an inconspicuous cutaneous angioma to be visualised more easily, as indicated by Doppman, Wirth, Di Chiro and Ommaya (1969).

Summary

1 The pathological findings in cases of spinal angioma are described. Deformed, atypical vessels with thickened walls are present over the surface of the cord, and some may be occluded by thrombus. The cord itself may be swollen or shrunken, and microscopic examination reveals neuronal degeneration, axonal demyelination, reactive gliosis and an apparent proliferation of small vessels, some of which may be thrombosed. Areas of infarction or haemorrhage may also be found, and if the angioma is intramedullary a localised collection of abnormal arteries, veins and sinusoidal vascular channels is present.

2 The manner in which the angioma causes a disturbance of cord function is uncertain, but it is suggested that the anomalous ateriovenous shunt leads in turn to an increased intramedullary venous pressure and reduced arteriovenous pressure gradient, thereby reducing intramedullary blood flow and causing ischaemia of the cord. This slowing of the intramedullary circulation will also lead to intravascular thrombosis, which enhances cord ischaemia. Other concepts which have previously been advanced to account for the development of symptoms in patients with these malformations are critically reviewed.

3 The clinical features of spinal angiomas are tentatively interpreted in terms of their pathology and suggested pathophysiology.

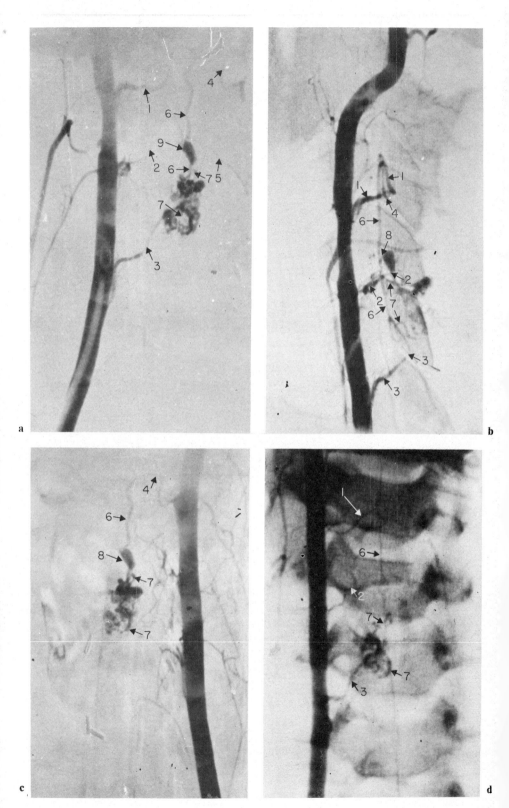

Chapter 11
Radiological investigations

B.E. Kendall

Although spinal angiomas often present fairly characteristic clinical features suggesting a long lesion affecting several adjacent segments of the spinal cord, a firm pre-operative diagnosis depends on radiological procedures in the majority of cases. Moreover, an essential prerequisite of their surgical treatment is the angiographic determination of the exact level of the shunt, its relationship to the surface of the spinal cord, and the geography of its feeding arteries and those supplying the cord itself. These points are discussed in detail in this chapter.

Figure 11.1. A 30-year-old woman presented with subarachnoid haemorrhage from a cervical angioma in 1971. Part of the angioma was removed, but an intramedullary component was left *in situ*. Subarachnoid haemorrhage recurred in 1974 and was associated with acute quadriparesis.

Right vertebral angiogram (1974) (a), antero-posterior and (b), lateral projections; left vertebral angiogram (1974)—(c), antero-posterior projection. The anterior radiculo-medullary arteries (1, 2, 3, 4, 5) are clearly visible. The anterior spinal artery (6) is enlarged between the C3 and C5 levels. Two branches from it (7) pass through the cord to supply the angioma which is situated posteriorly within and on the surface of the cord at the C4–5 and C5 levels. An aneurysm (8) projects posteriorly and inferiorly from the anterior spinal artery at C4 level, and its neck is indicated by an arrow.

Right vertebral angiogram (1967)—(d), antero-posterior projection. The angioma was smaller, the anterior spinal artery was not enlarged and the aneurysm was not present.

Applied anatomy

Spinal angiography has convincingly demonstrated that the essential abnormality in spinal angiomas is an arterio-venous shunt. The arteries supplying the malformation are radiculo-pial or radiculo-medullary vessels, and these may be more tortuous and dilated than usual. It may be difficult to distinguish these arteries at angiography when they run to the posterior aspect of the cord, and in such circumstances they will be referred to as 'radicular' arteries. A saccular aneurysm is sometimes found on one of them, and this may be a more frequent source of haemorrhage than the angioma itself (Figure 11.1). Arteries which supply angiomas situated posteriorly in the thoracic region usually arise within two or three segments of the level of the shunt, but feeders to cervical, thoraco-lumbar and lumbar angiomas not infrequently have a longer intradural course.

The shunt itself may consist of either a complex network of vessels containing several fistulous communications (Figure 11.2), or a single connection in which the exact point of transition from artery to vein may be uncertain (Figure 11.3). The blood from the malformation passes either directly or through small intramedullary or surface veins, to the longitudinal coronal veins. These veins are the most conspicuous feature of the angioma at operation, and their encroachment into the subarachnoid space is the main cause of the vermiform defects which are found at myelography. Although they connect with the intercostal, ascending lumbar and cervical veins through the epidural and paravertebral plexuses and the intervertebral veins, this is usually not conspicuous at angiography; in contrast, the longitudinal veins are often opacified over a considerable length, and it may be possible to visualise the posterior fossa veins rostrally, or the iliac veins caudally. The direction of

Figure 11.2. A 16-year-old male with a progressive paraparesis of 4 years' duration.

Left 8th intercostal angiogram (a), antero-posterior projection, early arterial phase; (b), later phase; (c), lateral projection, early arterial phase; (d), later phase. This intercostal vessel supplies the artery of Adamkiewicz (1). The anterior spinal artery (2) supplies a shunt on the right postero-lateral aspect of the cord at T7 level through a branch (3) passing round the right side of the cord. The anterior spinal atery is enlarged to the T8 level, and at least one further branch (4) passes toward the right side at this level and appears to supply a second, more anterior shunt, but the precise anatomy is uncertain due to overlying veins filling from the higher one. Dilated veins ascend on the left side of the theca posteriorly (5), and descend on the anterior aspect (7). A large vein (6) joining the longitudinal veins is shown on the right side of the theca.

(e) Right 7th intercostal angiogram. A posterior 'radicular' artery (8) feeds the upper part of the angioma. The same ascending vein (5) is seen, but there are additional ones on its right side. The right 6th (10) and 8th (11) intercostal arteries are opacified through normal paraspinal anastomoses. A branch (9) of the 8th intercostal also feeds the malformation, and this was confirmed by selective injection.

(f) Right 10th intercostal angiogram. This vessel supplies a further shunt situated postero-laterally at T9–10 level.

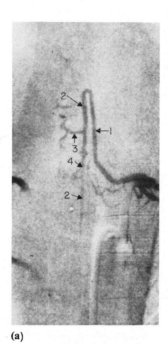

(a)

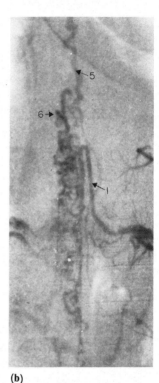

(b)

flow as visualised at angiography may be either rostral or caudal, and there is evidence to suggest that it varies with posture.

About 70 per cent of malformations are situated at or below the level of the 9th thoracic segment of the spinal cord, where they are located usually in the pia mater postero-laterally and are commonly supplied by a single posterior radiculo-pial artery. Only about 20 per cent of these caudally situated malformations have a significant intramedullary component; this component is easily recognised on angiograms if it is supplied by perforating branches of the anterior spinal artery, but its location within the cord may be more difficult or impossible to appreciate if it is fed by posterior radiculo-medullary arteries or by cruciate branches of the anterior spinal.

In the mid-thoracic region (4th–8th cord segments) malformations are often fed by two, or occasionally more, arteries which usually arise within three segments of each other. They may occur on any aspect of the cord but are usually posterior, and in some cases an intra-medullary component is present.

Malformations located between the 1st cervical and 3rd thoracic segments are frequently situated anteriorly, and very often are partly intramedullary. They are

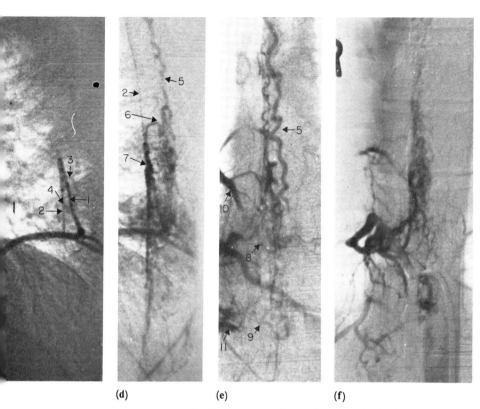

(d) (e) (f)

usually fed by several vessels, one of which is very often the anterior spinal artery or one of the arteries which supply it, and the rate of flow through them is usually faster than in more caudally placed lesions.

Plain X-rays

Plain X-rays of the spine usually show no significant abnormality. Occasionally, and more frequently in children than in adults, large arteriovenous channels may cause local widening of the spinal canal, but this may be found in association with any space-occupying lesion. Calcification has been described in the lesion in rare instances. The presence of other abnormalities such as a vertebral haemangioma or the radiological manifestation of Osler's disease may suggest the possibility of an underlying spinal angioma, but such associations are uncommon.

Routine chest X-ray may show abnormal dilatation of the azygos vein due to an increased blood flow through it, but this is rare.

Radio-isotope angiography

This may show regions of increased blood flow in the spinal canal, and thus help to localise vascular malforma-

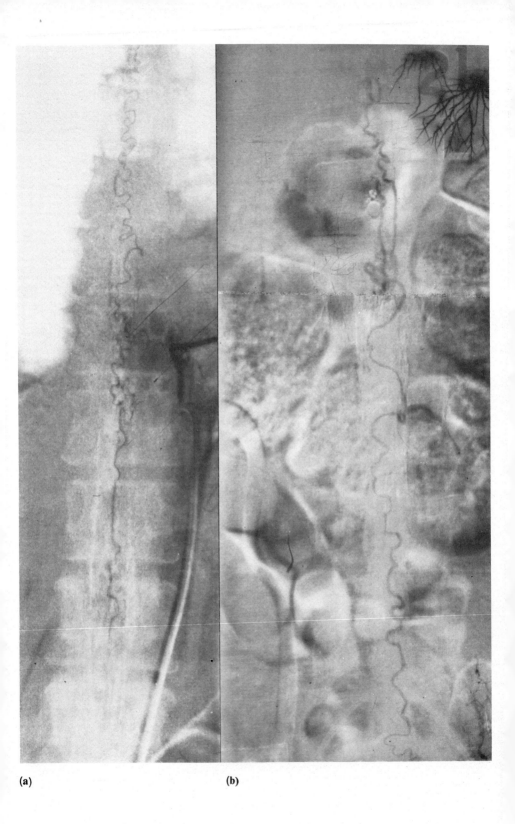

(a)

(b)

tions and tumours. Although it is not a routine procedure in most radiological departments, it may be helpful in rare cases in which a bruit over an expanded lumbar spinal canal suggests the presence of a large vascular lesion which may be injured by attempted lumbar puncture, and it may have some application in follow-up examinations after surgery. The method does not usually detect small angiomas and is, therefore, unlikely to be helpful in the investigation of patients with a progressive myelopathy in whom myelography shows no underlying cause (Di Chiro, Jones, Johnston and Allen, 1973).

Myelography

In most cases the diagnosis is made by myelography. The degree to which the abnormal vessels encroach into the subarachnoid space is variable, but it is not sufficient to allow reliable diagnosis with gas contrast. Moreover, gas myelography may cause changes in pressure which could precipitate haemorrhage.

Positive contrast is used routinely, and up to now iodophendylate myelography has been preferred. Since iodophendylate may react with blood and its breakdown products to cause pain and adhesive archnoiditis, it is not usually introduced until the cerebrospinal fluid is clear, even though it is removed routinely after the procedure. Some iodophendylate is frequently retained around the prominent vessels or between the adhesions which commonly exist in the vicinity of angiomas, and this may obscure detail on subsequent spinal angiograms. The introduction of safe water soluble agents, such as metrizamide, into routine practice will be a considerable advantage in this respect. It should be noted that a clinical deterioration may occur after iodophendylate myelography.

The angioma is best demonstrated when a sufficiently long segment of the theca has been filled with contrast to permit the relationship of the abnormal vessels to the circumference of the cord and the borders of the theca to be assessed. About 18 cc of myodil are usually sufficient for this purpose. The whole length of the theca is radiographed in both prone and supine positions, supplemented by oblique views if further detail is required. When the cervical region is abnormal the posterior fossa cisterns are also examined.

FACING PAGE
Figure 11.3. (a) A 50-year-old woman with an advancing paraparesis and a disturbance of micturition of several years' duration. Left 9th intercostal angiogram (antero-posterior projection). A posterior "radicular" artery feeds an angioma on the left side of the cord, from which veins ascend and descend. A normal "blush" in the left side of the 9th thoracic vertebral body is seen.
(b) A 25-year-old man with a paraparesis and right-sided sciatica for 4 months. Left internal iliac angiogram (antero-posterior projection). A tortuous, intrathecal vessel fills from a lateral sacral artery and ascends to the L1 vertebral level where it widens slightly before becoming convoluted at the T12 level. Two veins ascend from this region; the fistula is proximal and probably close to their origin, but its precise position is uncertain. (The photograph is a composite of 2 films, and the join is visible.)

Figure 11.4. (a) Same patient as in Figure 11.3(a). Myelogram (thoracic region, supine, postero-anterior projection). Typical tortuous defects due to the distended veins draining an angioma.

(b) A 19-year-old woman with a progressive paraparesis of 8 years' duration. Myelogram (lumbar region, semi-erect, antero-posterior projection). Marked vermiform defects caused by the enlarged intrathecal vessels associated with an angioma. The left 5th lumbar and the sacral root sheaths, and most of the subarachnoid space below S1 level are occluded by the mass of vessels, or by adhesions.

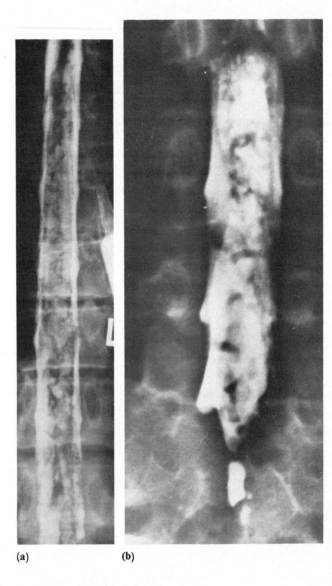

(a) (b)

Characteristic abnormality

The characteristic abnormality consists of vermiform defects in the column of contrast material, without any obstruction in the subarachnoid space (Figure 11.4). These defects may be localised to two or three segments, or may extend the whole length of the spinal canal and beyond it into the posterior fossa cisterns. In the thoracic regions they are usually most evident on the posterior aspect of the cord and theca, and are best seen or may only be shown on the supine films. Larger defects may also be found and are due to aneurysmal expansion of veins.

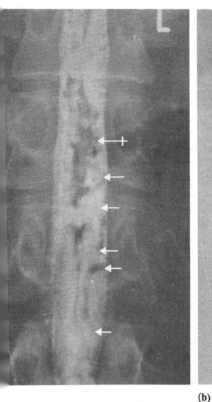 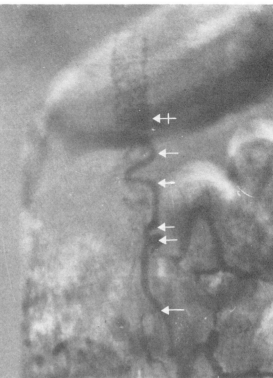

(b)

Figure 11.5. A 42-year-old man with progressive paraparesis and sensory loss for 2 years.

(a) Myelogram (lower) thoracic and upper lumbar region, supine, postero-anterior projection). A tortuous vessel (→) ascends from the left side of the theca at L1 to a nodular opacity blending with the left side of the cord at T11 (→).

(b) Angiogram of left 1st lumbar artery (antero-posterior projection, arterial phase) which supplies the posterior "radicular" artery (→) corresponding to the vessel indicated on the myelogram; this, in turn, supplies the shunt (→) which is at the site of the nodular defect on the myelogram. Convoluted draining veins are filled above this level.

Reproduced by courtesy of The Editor, *Excerpta Medica*.

Although it is not possible to localise the site of the shunt with certainty from the myelographic appearances, it is often situated near the level of the maximal venous distension. In about 25 per cent of patients the vascular impressions converge on one point, where a smooth projection from the cord is sometimes seen (Figure 11.5). Subsequent angiographic studies have indicated that this site usually corresponds with the position of the arterio-venous fistula itself. In a few cases, it may also be possible to recognise a feeding artery extending beside a nerve root from the side of the theca towards the cord (Figure 11.6). This is most often observed in the lumbar region, where the artery tends to have a long and tortuous intradural course. The size of the anterior spinal artery and the position of the anterior radiculo-medullary arteries may also be shown. All these features are helpful in the planning of spinal angiography.

The characteristic myelographic appearance of a spinal angioma may be simulated by other lesions, and in particular by vascular tumours with prominent draining veins. This is most likely to occur with haemangioblastomas, but the tumour usually causes a focal nodular expansion. If the only myelographic abnormality consists of an enlarged, tortuous segment of the anterior spinal artery, especially in the cervical and upper thoracic regions (Figure 11.7), the possibility of an underlying coarctation of the aorta should be considered. The appearance of normal, slightly tortuous veins, which are shown not infrequently over two or three segments,

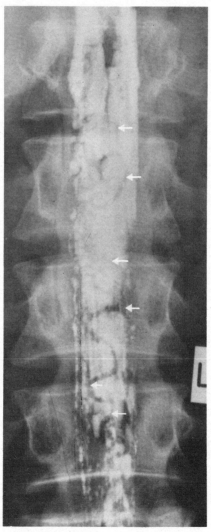

Figure 11.6. Same patient as Figure 11.3(b). Myelogram (lumbar region, supine, postero-anterior projection). The upper part of the vessel (→) ascending from the sacral region to the malformation at about the T12 level is clearly outlined.

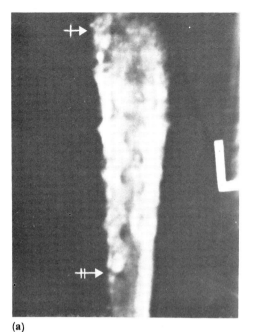

(a) (b)

Figure 11.7. A 13-year-old boy with a ventriculo-atrial shunt for hydrocephalus due to aqueduct stenosis. Coarctation of the aorta corrected when aged 11 years, following which he developed an increasing spastic quadriparesis and neurogenic intermittent claudication.

(a) Myelogram (lower cervical and upper thoracic region, prone, antero-posterior projection). A tortuous, dilated segment of the anterior spinal artery is seen between the 6th cervical and 4th thoracic levels. Enlarged segmental vessels extend from the right side of the theca at the 6th cervical (⇸) and 4th thoracic levels (⇻) to the anterior spinal artery.

A thoracic aortogram showed that there was residual coarctation at the usual site, distal to the left subclavian artery.

(b) Right subclavian angiogram (arterial phase, antero-posterior projection). Two anterior radiculo-medullary branches (→) from the right deep cervical artery fill the dilated segments of the anterior spinal artery (⇸), from which the right 3rd and 4th intercostal arteries fill retrogradely, as, in turn, does their common trunk (⇻) which leads to the aorta below the coarctation.

Reproduced by courtesy of the Editor, *Journal of Neurosurgery*.

especially posteriorly in the thoracic region, should not be mistaken for that of an angioma. Defects due to arachnoid trabecula branching from the septum posticum (Figure 11.8) are most prominent close to the midline; they can usually be traced to the longitudinal linear defect of the septum itself, and their pattern tends to be angular rather than serpiginous. An angioma may also be simulated on superficial examination by globulated iodophendylate, but any doubt is resolved by repeating the study. The appearance of tortuous lumbar nerve roots can usually be distinguished from that of an angioma by tracing their course into the root sheaths, but any doubt can be resolved by examining the spine in slight flexion to straighten them. Metastatic deposits

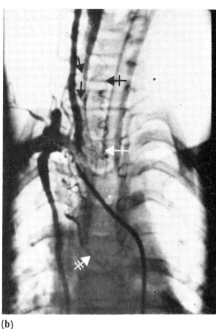

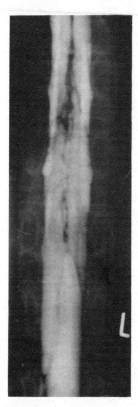

Figure 11.8. Patient with proven lower lumbar disc but no other abnormality. Myleogram (lower thoracic and upper lumbar region, supine, postero-anterior projection). Typical septum posticum. Note the irregular thickness of the central radiolucent band; septa passing laterally and downward from it at acute angles are due to arachnoid trabeculae.

on lumbar roots usually cause nodular defects which are unlike the tortuous defects seen in patients with an angioma.

Other features

Additional features may be present. Occasionally there is some swelling of the cord due usually to haemorrhage, oedema or an intramedullary component of the malformation (Figure 11.9), and if there is partial obstruction in such circumstances the appearances simulate those of an intramedullary tumour with associated venous distension (Figure 11.10). Not infrequently there is 'pocketing' of contrast medium (Figure 11.4b) by arachnoidal adhesions which have probably resulted from previous small haemorrhages; partial obstruction may result and, if the contrast medium is confined away from the malformation or the complex shadows of arachnoiditis disguise those due to the distended veins, the myelographic findings, though abnormal, will not be diagnostic.

It is difficult to ascertain the frequency with which all the myelographic features described above are absent in patients with a spinal angioma. Djindjian, Hurth and Houdart (1970) found that the myelographic appearance was characteristic in only about half of the patients in their series, although it was atypically abnormal in many of the remainder, and this accords with the experience of Teng and Papatheodorou (1964). The author, however, has no personal experience of any patient with a verified angioma in whom myelography, performed satisfactorily, failed to reveal abnormal appearances which could be related to the malformation.

Di Chiro and Wener (1973) discussed the limitations of myelography, recommending angiography in every patient with an obscure progressive disturbance of spinal cord function regardless of the myelographic findings. The author has investigated only 6 patients with a suspected angioma and negative myelogram by selective spinal angiography, but in each case no abnormality was shown.

Angiography

This is performed with several important aims in mind. Firstly, the level and extent of the shunting, its complexity, and its position in relation to the circumference of the spinal cord must be assessed. Secondly, the origin and course of the arteries feeding the malformation, their site of entry into it, and the presence of any coexisting arterial abnormalities such as an aneurysm (Figure 11.1), must be determined. Thirdly, the anterior radiculo-medullary and anterior spinal arteries to the segment of the cord related to the malformation must be visualised. This information is essential to the rational planning of corrective surgery.

AORTOGRAPHY

Mid-stream aortography rarely shows the cord vascula-ture in sufficient detail to assess the above features, especially in adults, and frequently fails to outline the malformation, particularly when the flow of blood through it is slow. Di Chiro (1972) has studied the effects of pressor amine potentiation and abdominal compression during aortography and has not found significant improvement in the visualisation of spinal cord arteries in man. Di Chiro, Doppman and Ommaya (1967) have also demonstrated that mid-stream aorto-graphy, in which concentrated contrast medium may enter all the vessels supplying the abnormal segment of spinal cord and perfuse it for a variable period, carries a greater risk of inducing neurological complica-tions than carefully conducted selective angiography.

SPINAL ANGIOGRAPHY

In this selective technique the orifices of the arteries supplying the appropriate radiculo-pial and radiculo-medullary arteries are injected with the contrast medium. The technique has been described in detail by Djindjian, Hurth and Houdart (1970) and by Doppman, Di Chiro and Ommaya (1969) and will be discussed only briefly. Local anaesthesia is preferred by the latter because this permits any deterioration in the patient's condition to be determined immediately. It is technically more satis-factory and more comfortable for the patient, however, to use general anaesthesia as preferred by Djindjian and his colleagues, who also cover the procedure with steroids in an attempt to minimise any neurological complications.

Unless there is a contra-indication, the author prefers to use general anaesthesia with muscular paralysis in order to provide good conditions for obtaining films suitable for subtraction. As in all angiography, the precise technique adopted will depend on the preferences of the individual radiologist. Various shapes of catheter,

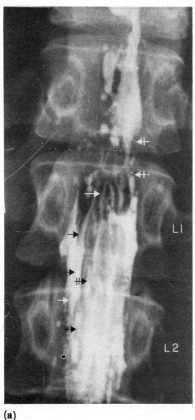

(a)

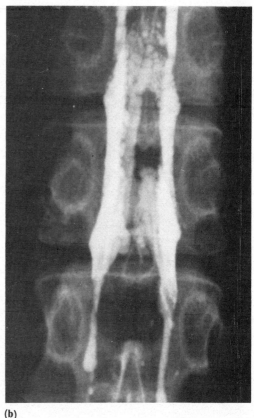

(b)

and the use of catheter deflectors and steering devices have been recommended, but an opaque PE 160 catheter with a cobra curve is usually adequate for an entire study.

Meglumine iothalamate (Conray 280) is used throughout the procedure. Three to 4 ml are injected into each of the normal segmental arteries in order to outline its posterior branch which supplies the paraspinal muscles and corresponding hemi-vertebra, and gives rise to radiculo-pial and/or radiculo-medullary branches. An injection is considered to be satisfactory only when a capillary blush is shown in the hemi-vertebra, and it may be necessary to repeat it after repositioning the catheter tip if this does not occur. When the artery supplying a malformation is located, it can safely be reinjected with 10 ml of contrast medium provided that it does not also supply the cord itself.

Three films are exposed at 3 second intervals in the exploratory study. The mode of filming necessary to show the malformation varies with the rate of flow through it. In general, films exposed at 2 second intervals

Figure 11.9. A 33-year-old housewife with intermittent left sciatica, and a paraparesis and disturbance of micturition of acute onset (Case 10, Appendix).
(a) and (b) Myelogram (lower thoracic and upper lumbar region, supine, postero-anterior projection). Linear opacity (→) due to posterior "radicular" artery ascending along right side of theca at L1 and L2 levels, with a tortuous vein (⇻) medial to it. The artery crosses to supply the malformation (↔) on the left postero-lateral aspect of the cord at the T12–L1 level. The cord is swollen at this level, and the findings at surgery suggested that an intramedullary component of the malformation was present.
(c) Selective angiogram of right 2nd lumbar artery (arterial phase, anteroposterior projection). Its posterior "radicular" artery (→) is shown supplying the malformation (↔). The veins are faintly outlined.

Reproduced by courtesy of the Editor, *Journal of Neurology, Neurosurgery and Psychiatry*.

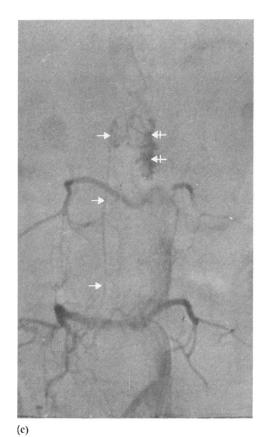

(c)

for 10 seconds are sufficient, but if the flow is slow, tortuous veins may not be fully outlined unless filming is continued at a slower rate for about 30 seconds.

Hazards

The procedure carries a small risk of sensitivity to the contrast medium as well as the risks of any arterial catheterisation procedure. Selective injections into the arteries supplying the spinal cord have caused a transient neurological deterioration in 5 of the 33 patients with angiomatous malformations submitted to 38 selective studies by the author; there was an increase in sphincter disturbance in 2 cases, in leg weakness in one, in weakness and sphincter disturbance in one; and in weakness, sensory and sphincter disturbances in the other. In all cases, the deterioration was both mild and transient, and similar reports of the safety of carefully conducted selective procedures are published by Djindjian, Hurth and Houdart (1970) and Di Chiro and Wener (1973).

Procedure

Clinical or myelographic findings determine which vessels are first injected. When a vessel feeding the angioma is located, the position of the shunt is ascertained in antero-posterior and lateral views. If it lies posteriorly, is fed by a posterior radiculo-pial artery, and does not appear to penetrate the cord, sufficient information for the accurate siting of a laminectomy has been obtained. Depending upon the level of the shunt, however, the procedure should be continued as indicated below to obtain further information essential to the planning of corrective surgery.

1 If further feeding vessels are opacified from segmental arteries filled through the normal paravertebral anastomoses (Figure 11.2) or retrogradely from the malformation, presumably because of increased pressure within

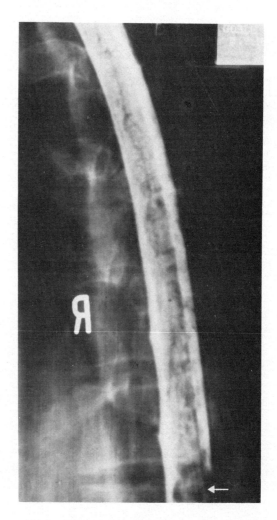

Figure 11.10. Myelogram (supine oblique, postero-anterior projection). Ependymoma causing swelling of conus medullaris (→) and considerable obstruction of the subarachnoid space. There are extensive, tortu-ous and dilated veins in the lower thoracic region, similar to those of an angioma.

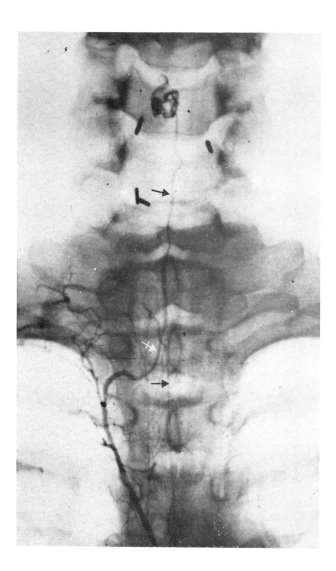

Figure 11.11. The same patient as Figure 11.1. Right superior aortic intercostal angiogram (arterial phase, antero-posterior projection). The anterior spinal artery (→) fills from an anterior radiculo-medullary artery (↦) up to the angioma at the C5 level, and supplies its lower part.

it during the injection, the segmental arteries supplying them should be injected.

2 When the malformation is located between the 1st cervical and 3rd thoracic segments of the cord, both vertebral arteries, the costo- and thyro-cervical trunks, and the upper four aortic intercostal arteries should be injected (Figure 11.11).

3 When it is situated between the 4th and 11th thoracic segments, the four intercostal arteries above and below those shown to be supplying the malformation, and the corresponding contralateral vessels, should be opacified.

4 When it lies below the 12th thoracic segment, the three segmental arteries above, and all the vessels at and below the level of the malformation on both sides should

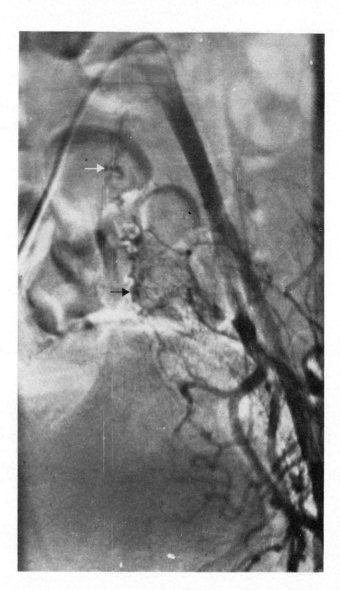

Figure 11.12. Same patient as Figure 11.4 (b) Left common iliac angiogram (arterial phase, antero-posterior projection; a later arterial phase has been used as a mask, and subtraction is imperfect due to movement). A tortuous branch (→) of a left lateral sacral artery is shown to be filled as high as the 5th lumbar vertebra; it is ascending towards a malformation situated more rostrally.

be injected, including the internal iliac arteries (Figure 11.12).

5 In all cases, care must be taken to define also the anterior radiculo-medullary vessels supplying the anterior spinal artery in the region of the angioma, for several reasons. Firstly, it often supplies the angioma when this is situated anteriorly on the surface of the cord, and occasionally it sends a circumferential branch to feed a posteriorly placed one (Figure 11.2). In addition, it often contributes to an intramedullary extension of the malformation (Figure 11.1), and may supply shunts in the region of the conus through its cruciate branches (Figure 11.13). Secondly, it is important to know the

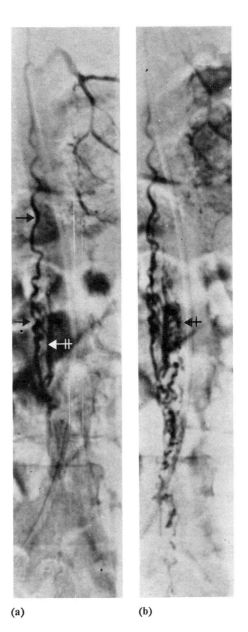

Figure 11.13. The same patient as Figure 11.4(b) and 11.12. Left 9th inter-costal angiogram, (a) arterial phase and (b) late arterial and venous phase, antero-posterior projec-tion. The artery of Adamkiewicz is outlined, and the enlarged anterior spinal artery (→) feeds a malformation (↠) on the left side of the conus through one of its cruciate branches (⊪→). Tortuous veins extend from this level, mainly inferiorly.

(a)   (b)

relationship of the blood supply of the cord to the propo-sed operative field. And thirdly, although it is uncommon for a major anterior radiculo-medullary artery to origi-nate from the same intercostal stem as an artery feeding the angioma, it is important to exclude this with certainty.

In the author's experience an angiographic study performed in the manner described will provide all the information essential for the further management of the patient, and a more extensive study is not strictly necessary and potentially more hazardous.

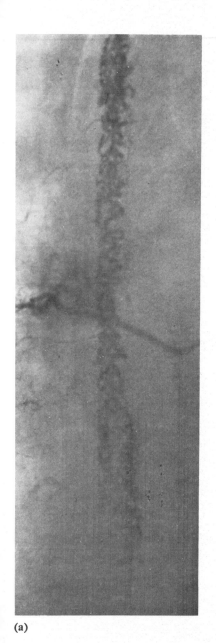

(a)

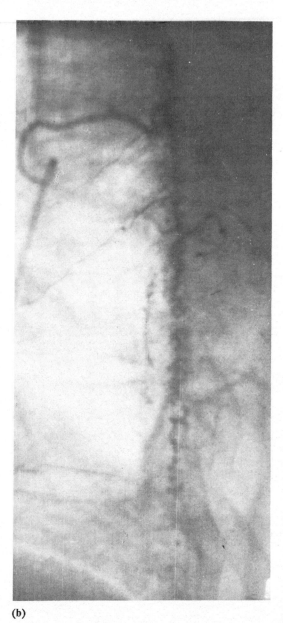

(b)

Ideally, angiography should be repeated following surgery in order to show that the aims of the operation have been achieved. At this time it is sufficient to opacify only the vessels previously shown to supply the malformation, the immediately adjacent ones, and the corresponding contralateral vessels.

Angiographic appearances

As already indicated, the shunt may be fed by a single

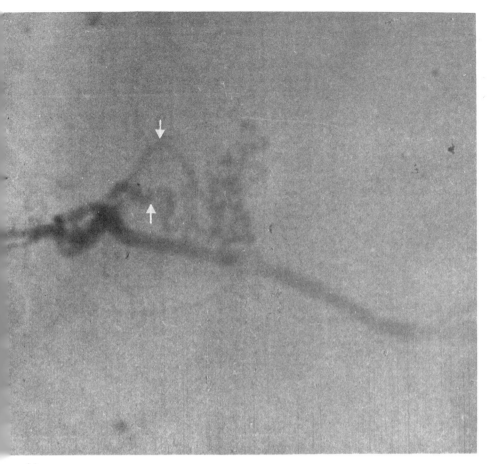

(c)

Figure 11.14. A 63-year-old man with progressive paraparesis and sensory loss in the legs for several years (Case 5, Appendix).

Right 6th intercostal angiogram, (a) antero-posterior and (b) lateral projections. An extensive convoluted mass of draining veins, mainly on the posterior aspect of the cord, hides the shunt.

(c) Same patient, early arterial phase, antero-posterior projection. The posterior "radicular" branch of the intercostal artery can now be seen to split into 2 branches (→) which run a somewhat tortuous horizontal course to the right side of the cord and then converge on the shunt. The proximal parts of the draining veins are outlined.

artery or by several, and the drainage may be through a single coiled longitudinal vein or through two or more veins. In children or young adults, the arterial supply is more often multiple, draining veins are usually more rapidly opacified and contrast medium tends to be cleared relatively faster than in older patients.

The extent and complexity of the angiomatous vessels filled on a selective angiogram varies, but often the intertwining or overlapping of coiled veins on later films of a series makes detailed analysis impossible (Figure 11.14). The early films are of crucial importance

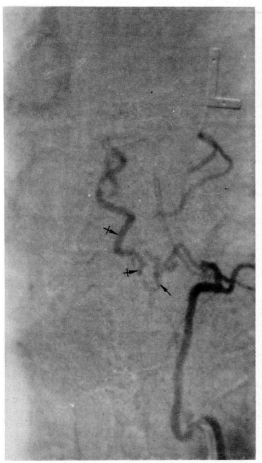
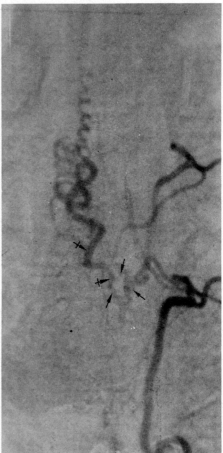

(a)   (b)

Figure 11.15. A 55-year-old man with weakness and numbness in the legs for 6 weeks.
Left 5th intercostal angiogram, antero-posterior projection, (a) early arterial and (b) later phase. The posterior "radicular" artery divides into tortuous branches (→) which shunt into a wider vein (↦). This drains superiorly before dividing into convoluted ascending and descending veins.

for visualisation of the shunt. It is at the site where feeding arteries converge (Figure 11.15), and at or proximal to where the draining veins diverge (Figure 11.16). A single posterior 'radicular' artery may give off two branches which converge on a shunt, or branches may converge from different segmental arteries and be seen to progress to the same point by comparison with the respective selective angiograms. The pattern of venous filling from an individual shunt is constant; accordingly, if there is more than one feeding artery, the position of the shunt can be determined by tracing this identical venous pattern back to it (Figure 11.2). This procedure is followed on antero-posterior and lateral views for each feeder in order to plot the precise position and extent of the shunt, and to exclude the presence of more than one region of shunting, which is an uncommon occurrence. When there is a single feeding artery and solitary draining vein there may be difficulty in localising precisely the site of the shunt itself (Figure 11.3b), but there is often some widening in the course of such a vessel in the region where it changes from artery to vein. For practical purposes, such a vessel should be excised in the proximal part of its course, to ensure removal of both feeder and shunt.

Summary

1 Plain X-rays of the spine usually show no significant abnormality in patients with a spinal angioma.
2 In most cases, a spinal angioma is diagnosed by positive contrast myelography, which should be performed in both prone and supine positions. The characteristic abnormality consists of vermiform defects without

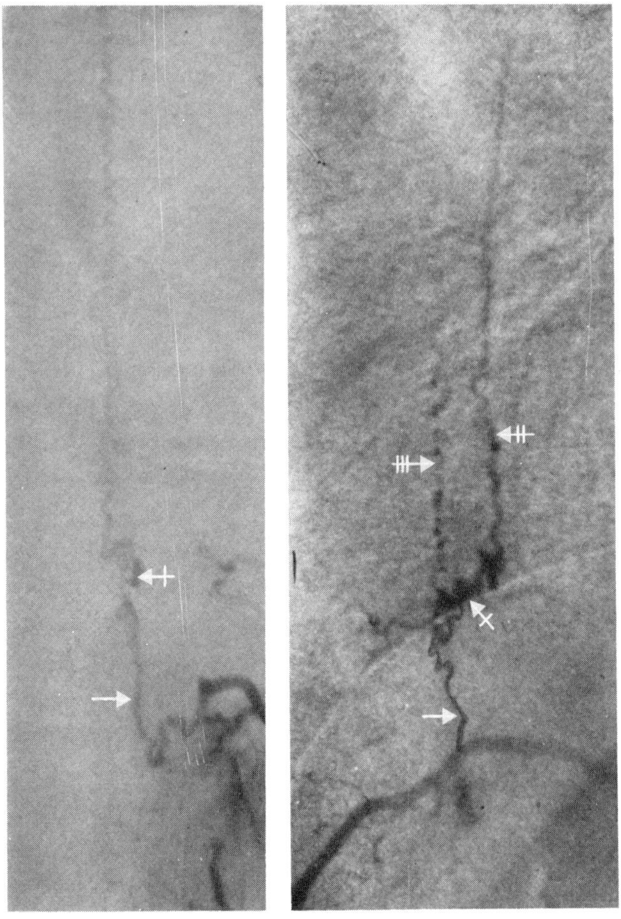

(a) **(b)**

Figure 11.16. A 40-year-old man with a progressive paraparesis for several years.

Left 10th intercostal angiogram, (a), antero-posterior and (b), lateral projection. The posterior "radicular" branch (→) extends along the left side of the cord to the shunt (+>) at the T11 level. In the lateral view a tortuous vein ascends on the anterior (++>) and another on the posterior aspect (+++>) of the cord. These are superimposed on the antero-posterior view.

obstruction to the subarachnoid space, and it is sometimes possible to recognise the probable site of the shunt, and the position of arteries feeding it. Additional features, such as swelling of the cord or partial obstruction, may also be found.

3 Selective spinal angiography is performed in order to delineate the level, morphology and extent of the arteriovenous fistula, the origin of its feeding arteries and the blood supply to the related segment of the cord. Brief technical and procedural details are provided, the hazards of the procedure are discussed, and the angiographic appearances of spinal angiomas are reviewed.

Chapter 12
Surgical treatment

There is no satisfactory medical treatment of spinal angiomas. Occasional cases have been encountered in which anticoagulant drugs were prescribed in the belief that symptoms were due to intravascular thrombosis, but such treatment is clearly contra-indicated in a condition known to be associated with subarachnoid and intramedullary haemorrhage. Radiotherapy has sometimes been given, but there is little clinical evidence that it provides any benefit in the majority of cases (Kaplan, Roswit and Krueger, 1952; Krayenbühl and Yaşargil, 1963).

Before the advent of selective angiography the surgical treatment of spinal angiomas was also unsatisfactory, because the relative importance of individual vessels to the normal spinal circulation, and their relationship to the anomalous arteriovenous shunt, could seldom be appreciated at operation, and their 'blind' excision, coagulation or ligation was often associated with a deterioration rather than an improvement in the condition of patients. As a consequence many neurologists and neurosurgeons came to regard these lesions as inoperable and confined their attention to helping patients prepare for a life of permanent invalidism. However, now that it is possible to delineate the arteries feeding the angioma and the cord, and the precise topography of the malformation itself, the aims of surgery can be defined and achieved more easily, and a gratifying degree of improvement can be expected in many patients after operation. Surgical treatment is planned with the aim of occluding the blood supply to the malformation, and preventing its revascularisation.

Indications for treatment

Patients may remain asymptomatic for many years, but once leg weakness or a disturbance of gait has started to develop, the daily activities and capabilities of most will become increasingly restricted, and many will ultimately become severely disabled unless the malformation is treated. In some cases progression occurs very rapidly, but in others symptoms advance much more slowly and disability may not become restrictive for many years, if at all. This poses a difficult problem because on the one hand surgical treatment carries a definite risk of damage to the cord, and on the other there is the risk of a sudden, severe exacerbation of symptoms, or subarachnoid haemorrhage may occur, if the malformation is left untreated; moreover, the degree of irreversible damage to the cord may slowly increase if there is any delay in treatment, thereby reducing the extent of ultimate functional recovery after operation. Although every case must be assessed individually, certain generalisations can justifiably be made.

If an asymptomatic angioma is an incidental finding during the course of investigations performed for other reasons, the malformation is probably best left undisturbed unless it subsequently leads to the development of symptoms.

In patients with mild symptoms and no incapacity, the advisability of treatment depends upon an assessment of the risks of surgery, which will relate to the general condition of the patient, the experience of the surgeon, the availability of angiographic facilities and of such technical aids as the operating microscope, and the characteristics of the malformation as indicated by angiography In the author's view, however, surgery should usually be considered at any early stage, for the prospects for complete recovery are greater at that time.

When feasible, surgery is probably indicated in all patients with symptoms that are progressing rapidly or with functional incapacity necessitating a change in the normal pattern of daily life. It is similarly indicated in all patients who have had a subarachnoid haemorrhage, even if complete recovery has occurred, because of the risks of re-bleeding.

Feasibility of treatment

The feasibility of surgical treatment and the manner in which this can be achieved most satisfactorily depends on the location of the malformation and the source of its blood supply.

POSTERIORLY SITUATED, EXTRAMEDULLARY ANGIOMAS

In about 80 per cent of cases the angioma is mainly or completely extramedullary, is posterior to the cord, and is fed by vessels which either fail to supply the cord at all or contribute only to the posterior spinal circulation. In such circumstances the vessels feeding it can be occluded, and the main mass of the malformation can be removed if desired; abnormal vessels sometimes penetrate the cord, but these can be divided and left undisturbed. Angiomas in this site may be fed by branches which come from the front of the cord, and these can usually be occluded with impunity, even in the uncommon instance when they originate from vessels supplying the anterior spinal artery.

ANTERIORLY SITUATED AND/OR
INTRAMEDULLARY ANGIOMAS

About 20 per cent of angiomas are situated mainly anterior to, and/or within the cord, and are difficult to treat because of their inaccessibility. Moreover, such angiomas are more likely to be fed by the anterior spinal artery or one of its feeding vessels, occlusion of which may lead to further damage to the cord. The feasibility of surgery in such circumstances is best considered by reference to specific situations which well exemplify the general problems. The total removal of angiomas situated mainly or completely within the cord has occasionally been reported, but this procedure is particularly hazardous, is usually unnecessary, and will receive no further consideration here.

Cervical and upper thoracic angiomas

Angiomas situated above the 2nd or 3rd thoracic segment often surround the cord or are situated anterior to it, are usually fed from several sources and very frequently are intramedullary, at least in part. Until recently they were usually considered to be inoperable, and certainly their complete removal is generally not feasible. It may be possible, however, to ligate intra- or extradurally any feeders which are accessible (Houdart, Djindjian and Hurth, 1966; Bailey and Sperl, 1969), and inaccessible feeders can sometimes be occluded by embolisation (Djindjian, Cophignon, Rey, Théron, Merland and Houdart, 1973), or extravertebral ligation in the neck (Logue, Aminoff and Kendall, 1974). Such procedures are usually well tolerated even if some of the occluded vessels previously supplied the anterior spinal artery, presumably because the latter is fed by several radiculo-medullary vessels in this region. Nevertheless, following such procedures one of the patients described by Bailey and Sperl (1969) was left with a partially paralysed arm, and a patient briefly referred to by Djindjian and his colleagues (1973) became quadriplegic, although his condition began to improve a few weeks later.

Experience in the treatment of cervical angiomas is still very limited, and although the potential hazards are clearly evident, it is not yet possible to make any useful assessment of the morbidity rate. Accordingly, since most of these malformations are situated anteriorly, and several or all of their feeding vessels may be contributing to the anterior spinal circulation, the author considers that in this region no more than one major feeder should be occluded at any one time, unless it is certain that additional ones do not supply the normal circulation. This will necessitate a multi-stage procedure to obliterate the blood supply of most of these angiomas, but this seems unavoidable in the interests of safety.

Present techniques do not permit the safe occlusion of feeding vessels when—as sometimes occurs—they arise from the anterior spinal artery itself. It is rare for the latter to constitute the sole source of supply to an angioma, however, and occlusion of coexisting segmental feeders may be of some benefit in reducing both the risk of subarachnoid haemorrhage and the rate of advance of symptoms by diminishing the volume of the shunt, even though the angioma remains partly vascularised and the supply from the remaining feeders may increase.

Angiomas fed by the artery of Adamkiewicz

No satisfactory treatment for angiomas fed directly by the anterior spinal artery is available at present, but the development of new microsurgical techniques may permit this in the future. The treatment of malformations supplied partly or wholly by the artery of Adamkiewicz is controversial. Although there is a natural reluctance to occlude a vessel which seems also to be the major feeder of the anterior spinal artery, experimental and clinical studies suggest that to do so may not lead to the catastrophic outcome that might have been anticipated.

Fried, Di Chiro and Doppman (1969) ligated the angiographically defined artery of Adamkiewicz in 10 Rhesus monkeys who were sacrificed between 4 and 10 days later, when post-mortem confirmation of complete occlusion was obtained; motor function was normal in 5 and minimally impaired in the remainder, suggesting that enough blood could flow down the anterior spinal artery to prevent serious ischaemia of the cord. In another 9 monkeys the anterior spinal was ligated above the point where it was fed by the artery of Adamkiewicz, and this also was well tolerated, suggesting that the artery of Adamkiewicz could itself provide sufficient blood to meet the requirements of the lumbar cord. However, when the anterior spinal was ligated below the entrance of this artery, 7 of 11 monkeys became paraplegic, 2 lost the ability to stand and 1 could only stand with support, while the remaining animal became only slightly disabled. Thus, when both sources of blood supply to the lumbo-sacral cord were obstructed severe damage resulted, but occlusion of one was well tolerated. After reviewing some of the previously published clinical case reports, these authors concluded that insufficient evidence was available to attribute cord infarction solely to occlusion of the artery of Adamkiewicz, for most cases were complicated by additional factors which would have diminished blood flow to the cord from other sources.

In patients with a spinal angioma, several observations also suggest that the artery of Adamkiewicz can sometimes be occluded with impunity. Newton and Adams (1968) treated the angioma in a 22-year-old paraplegic by embolising both of its feeders, one of which was the artery of Adamkiewicz, and the patient regained a useful amount of power in the legs. Occlusion of this artery was also well tolerated in 3 cases reported by Di Chiro and Wener (1973). In contrast, however, Djindjian and his colleagues found that leg weakness was increased after its accidental ligation in a patient with an intramedullary angioma supplied by it, and have deliberately avoided such a procedure unless the patient is already paraplegic.

Insufficient information is currently available to permit firm conclusions to be reached with regard to the treatment of patients who are mildly disabled. In those who have been severely disabled for at least 3 months, embolic occlusion of the artery of Adamkiewicz when this vessel is feeding an underlying angioma, is justified if little further deterioration can occur, but some recovery may result.

In an attempt to find a more satisfactory solution, Djindjian and his colleagues (1973) have recently attempted to occlude selectively with small gelfoam emboli those of its branches which feed the malformation, provided that the parent vessel is large. They have also studied new methods of approach to the anterior surface of the cord and are developing a microsurgical technique to ligate, after myelocommissurotomy, those sulco-commissural arteries which feed intramedullary angiomas from the artery of Adamkiewicz—anterior spinal axis. Such techniques cannot be evaluated, however, until further experience with them has accumulated.

Methods of treatment

There is good general agreement that decompressive procedures confer therapeutic benefit, usually slight and short-lived, in less than one-fifth of cases, while the clinical condition of the remainder is either unchanged or worse after operation (cf. Newman, 1959; Krayenbühl and Yaşargil, 1963; Luessenhop and Dela Cruz, 1969). Similarly, the attempted removal, ligation or coagulation of major vessels whose nature has not been defined radiologically has often led to disappointing results. This might have been anticipated since, without the aid of angiography, it is often difficult to determine the most appropriate site for laminectomy, and the 'blind' ligation or excision of all the exposed vessels on the surface of the cord does not necessarily ensure removal of the abnormal arteriovenous communication and may damage vessels supplying the cord itself.

It is unnecessary to review all the earlier reports on treatment, but three recent ones require comment before the angiographically-guided treatment of these malformations is discussed. Shephard (1963, 1965) systematically treated 11 patients by excision of abnormal vessels on the surface of the cord after laminectomy which seems to have been guided by the clinical and myelographic findings, and sometimes involved as many as 8 or 9 vertebrae. Angiography provided some information about the site of the malformation in one case, but it is likely that in most—if not all—of the others it was not performed at all, so that the abnormal communication between arteries and veins was not necessarily removed. Although 8 patients were considered to have done moderately or very well after operation, insufficient data were provided for independent assessment, and in 2 of these cases symptoms subsequently recurred. The importance of this study, however, is the general conclusions that it enabled Shephard to reach at a time when these malformations were usually considered to be inoperable, for he suggested that their surgical treatment was more feasible than had previously been appreciated, emphasising that their blood supply was usually separate from that of the cord and that the presence of a significant intramedullary component was relatively uncommon.

More recently Krayenbühl, Yaşargil and McClintock (1969) reported the results of surgical excision in 17 patients, but again their use of angiography appears to have been limited. Excision was facilitated by the use of the operating microscope, after laminectomy which often extended over 6 or more vertebrae, and total removal was attempted unless there was an intramedullary extension or the abnormal vessels on the surface of the cord extended over too great a length. It seems probable, therefore, that the abnormal communication between arterial and venous systems was often removed, at least in those cases in which abnormal vessels were followed and excised throughout their rostro-caudal extent. The result of surgery could not be assessed in one patient because insufficient time had elapsed since operation, and in 2 others the absence of any significant pre-operative deficit makes assessment impossible. Improvement, often considerable, occurred in 11 of the remaining 14 patients, but the length of postoperative follow-up was not indicated, so that full evaluation of these results is difficult.

In the belief that symptoms are due to diversion of blood from the normal supply to the cord, the veins draining an angioma have sometimes been ligated in an attempt to obstruct flow through the anomalous arteriovenous shunt and redirect it into normal channels, thereby increasing the supply to the ischaemic cord (Chatterjee and Roy, 1968; Chatterjee, 1969). As indicated in Chapter 10, however, it is unlikely that 'steal' of blood from the normal spinal circulation is the usual cause of symptoms, and the benefit which sometimes appears to have followed this procedure was probably due to retrograde thrombosis of vessels feeding the malformation. Moreover, the procedure might well increase the risk of haemorrhage by causing an increased intraluminal pressure proximal to the obstruction, and in a case reported by Kaufman, Ommaya, Di Chiro and Doppman (1970) subarachnoid haemorrhage did indeed occur a few weeks after the 'blind' ligation of a large extradural vein.

The logical treatment of spinal angiomas is to occlude their blood supply when this is feasible, and now that the arteries feeding them can be defined and distinguished pre-operatively from those supplying the cord, this can be achieved in several ways. It must be noted, however, that in exceptional cases the appearance of the angioma at operation may be markedly dissimilar to that anticipated from the findings at angiography, usually because one of its feeding arteries has been occluded by thrombus and the malformation has not been fully outlined as a consequence. In the following discussion reference has been confined when possible to large individual series of cases in the interest of brevity and to permit adequate assessment of the results achieved.

In general, this procedure is technically simpler than those in which the malformation is excised and requires less handling of the cord. Moreover, it can sometimes be used in the treatment of anteriorly situated angiomas and of those which are partly or completely intra-medullary.

Proximal ligation

Houdart, Djindjian and Hurth (1966) reported clinical improvement in 2 of 3 patients with a thoracic angioma after ligation of their source of supply at a point close to the origin of the intercostal arteries from the aorta, and shortly afterwards Baker, Love and Layton (1967) reported the successful treatment of 5 patients by transthoracic ligation and division of abnormal feeding vessels and the intercostal arteries from which they arose. The latter authors considered the transthoracic approach as sound as a direct one in the spinal canal, but there are good reasons for questioning this view. In particular, the former technique may permit revascu-larisation of the malformation from arteries in adjacent segments through collateral vessels forming part of the paravertebral anastomotic network.

Ligation within the spinal canal

This procedure necessitates a laminectomy centred on the site of the feeding vessels, but if successfully achieved makes it unlikely that revascularisation of the malforma-tion will occur through collateral channels. In some cases, however, vessels may enter the dura anteriorly rather than with the nerve roots, so that they are surgically inaccessible by this approach (Houdart, Djindjian and Hurth, 1966). It is sometimes difficult to recognise angiographically defined feeding arteries at operation, but in such circumstances it may be possible to locate them in the extradural space, where two or more arteries sometimes unite before penetrating the theca, as in one of the cases described in the Appendix (Case 13, p. 160).

If there are several feeders to the malformation, some authors do not ligate them all at the same operation, but Ommaya, Di Chiro and Doppman (1969) have preferred a one-stage procedure. These authors ligated all the feeders in 11 patients with an angioma in the thoracic or lumbar regions, and symptomatic improvement occurred in every case but one, in whom insufficient time had elapsed for adequate assessment; in 5 of these 11 cases there was a significant improvement in gait such that one patient, who had been virtually chair-bound for a year, subsequently recovered sufficiently well to get about with a crutch.

The drawback of this procedure is that the malformation will continue to be vascularised and may lead to further symptoms if feeders are unrecognised at angiography and/or operation, and are left undisturbed. In such circumstances the remaining feeder can always be ligated at a second operation provided that it is recognised at post-operative angiography, and for this reason it is wise to opacify not only the segmental arteries from which feeders were previously shown to arise, but also the immediately adjacent vessels and the corresponding ones on the other side.

Ligation of feeding arteries and excision of the fistula

In order to reduce still further the possibility of revascularisation of the malformation, the intradural ligation of its feeding vessels can be combined, when feasible, with excision of its fistulous portion. The response of 19 patients to this procedure was briefly reported by Djindjian, Houdart and Hurth (1969); there was no useful recovery in 7 who were completely paraplegic before operation, but the remaining 12 patients showed a variable degree of improvement which in 4 was sufficient to permit them to return to a normal way of life.

This procedure was also adopted in 15 of the 16 cases from the National Hospitals for Nervous Diseases summarised in the Appendix and which were previously reported by Logue, Aminoff and Kendall (1974). In 12 the malformation was defined by selective spinal angiography, and in another 2 it was visualised at aortography although its feeders could not be recognised. The findings at operation usually conformed well with the angiographic appearance, but in spite of this one of the segmental feeding vessels previously demonstrated could not be found in 3 cases, possibly because no extradural search was made. Temporary occlusion of feeders led to a diminution in bulk or pulsation of the malformation, and/or a darkening in colour of the blood within it in all but one of the 13 patients in whom this manoeuvre was performed; such changes were sometimes slow to develop, taking place over several minutes, but they were usually reversed very rapidly when the blood supply was restored.

In 3 patients the presence of an intramedullary component of the malformation was suspected because there was local swelling of the cord, with conspicuous vessels running from its surface to connect with the abnormal extramedullary vessels. This intramedullary component was left undisturbed, and probably accounted for the abrupt advance of symptoms which occurred in one of these patients 2 months after operation and continued until his death 3 years later.

The previously progressive downhill course of 14 patients was arrested by surgery and in 12 there was worthwhile improvement in gait. There was an improvement in disturbances of micturition in 7 patients, and in disorders of defaecation in 6. One patient became more incapacitated immediately after surgery, requiring the support of 2 sticks rather than his previous one to get about, but his condition has not deteriorated further since that time.

Embolisation of feeding vessels

In 1968 Doppman, Di Chiro and Ommaya reported the successful occlusion by percutaneous embolisation of the main vessel feeding a mid-thoracic angioma which could not be approached by laminectomy because of a large, overlying cutaneous angioma, and shortly afterwards Newton and Adams (1968) reported the treatment of another patient by a similar technique; in both cases undoubted clinical benefit followed the procedure. Since that time Doppman and his colleagues have gained further experience with this approach and in 1971 they reviewed the outcome in their first 7 patients; embolisation was successfully accomplished, under local anaesthesia, in 5 cases without any concomitant deterioration in cord function, and in 3 it was said to have been followed by progressive neurological improvement.

Occlusion was accomplished primarily with metal pellets, but muscle fragments and gelfoam were also introduced in the hope of promoting thrombosis. The angioma was defined angiographically, and the angiographic catheter was then replaced by a larger one to permit the introduction of pellets of sufficient size to occlude the feeding vessel. If the parietal branch of the segmental (intercostal or lumbar) artery was larger than the branch to the angioma, it was necessary to occlude it before smaller pellets would pass to the latter, but this caused only some mild, local discomfort. The aim of the procedure was to occlude the feeder within the spinal canal in order to prevent the development of a secondary supply to the angioma from adjacent segments via collateral vessels. Once this had been achieved, the segmental vessel from which it originated was also occluded with muscle fragments and gelfoam.

The technique has the merit of simplicity and safety compared with procedures necessitating laminectomy, but the length of follow-up is inadequate as yet to permit more detailed evaluation, particularly with regard to the permanence of vascular occlusion induced by this means. Nevertheless, it clearly has useful application in the treatment of patients when a direct approach is particularly hazardous or impractical because of advancing age, poor general condition, an anteriorly situated or mainly intramedullary malformation, or the presence of extensive arachnoiditis, and when operation has previously failed because the malformation could not be removed and its feeding arteries were not recognised. Moreover, if subsequent studies confirm its value, the procedure may well become the treatment of first choice, a more direct approach being reserved for those in whom the angioma cannot satisfactorily be obliterated by this means.

Summary

1 The indications for surgical treatment are reviewed and, when feasible, treatment is advised in all patients with functional incapacity, rapidly advancing symptoms or a history of subarachnoid haemorrhage. In patients with mild symptoms and no incapacity, the advisability of surgery depends on an assessment of its associated risks, and asymptomatic angiomas are best left undisturbed.

2 Most angiomas are situated posteriorly and are extramedullary, and their treatment therefore poses no special problems. The management of anteriorly situated and/or intramedullary malformations is more hazardous because of their inaccessibility and because their feeding vessels may be closely related to those supplying the cord, and is discussed in some detail.

3 The aim of treatment is to occlude the blood supply of the angioma and prevent its revascularisation. This can be achieved in several ways depending upon the position of the angioma and source of its feeding vessels as defined by angiography. Ligation of feeding vessels

·within the spinal canal is usually adequate, but concomitant excision of the fistulous portion of the malformation reduces the possibility of its revascularisation. Alternatively, feeding vessels can sometimes be occluded by percutaneous embolisation. The merits and disadvantages of these various procedures are discussed and the results of treatment reviewed. The progressive advance of symptoms is usually halted and in many cases worthwhile improvement follows.

Chapter 13
Practical aspects of surgical treatment

Valentine Logue

The views expressed in this chapter are based on the author's personal experience of a series of 16 cases treated by operation and followed up for a sufficient length of time (1–7 years, mean 3·1 years) to indicate the short- and medium-term results. In one of these cases, a patient with a cervical lesion, the operation was extra-spinal and involved ligation of the vessels of supply which arose from branches of the subclavian arteries, but the remaining 15 cases were explored intradurally. The results of surgery in this series have been summarised in the preceding chapter and by Logue, Aminoff and Kendall (1974), and need not be recapitulated here.

Principles of surgical treatment

The principles of treatment, and the factors on which they depend, are as follows:

1 The angiomatous circulation is usually distinct from that of the cord and its arterial component can be removed with little risk of ischaemia to the latter. Symptoms are probably due to a reduction of blood flow within the spinal cord because of a high intramedullary venous pressure (Aminoff, Barnard and Logue, 1974), rather than to 'steal' from the anterior or posterior spinal circulation as has sometimes been proposed. The arteries supplying the anterior spinal circulation, and in particular the artery of Adamkiewicz, only rarely contribute to the supply of angiomas situated below the cervical region (and did not do so in any of these 16 cases), a fact which can be demonstrated routinely at angiography.

2 In 80 per cent of cases the malformation is situated on the back of the spinal cord and is therefore easily accessible for surgical excision. Some of those which extend on to the antero-lateral aspect and receive branches from vessels supplying the anterior spinal artery may also be removable.

3 The precise demonstration of the arterial supply by selective catheterisation is essential. Except in the cervical region, the supply is usually via a single vessel, but if it is more extensive the vessels usually come from adjacent segments and sometimes unite extradurally to enter the theca as a single artery. An occasional exception to this arrangement is found among angiomas in the lumbo-sacral area, which may receive an additional, entirely separate supply by a vessel ascending from the sacral arteries.

4 (a) In determining the optimum site for exposure of

the main feeding vessel, reliance cannot be placed on the segmental level of neurological damage which may be several segments away from the main angiomatous area, as in 2 cases in this series.

(b) The myelographic visualisation of feeding vessels is unreliable. Although a large feeding artery, confirmed by angiography, may sometimes be recognisable near a nerve root, this is too uncommon to be of practical help, and in an extensive angioma even the differentiation of the arterial congerie from the venous drainage may be impossible.

5 The shunt must be removed in its entirety. At operation this area is distinguishable from the larger, straighter and darker veins emerging from it by its arterialised nature and characteristic 'coiling'. Although good results have been achieved in the treatment of these angiomas by simple clipping or ligation intradurally of the main feeding vessel without excision of the malformation itself, experience with malformations in other situations has shown that unless the fistulous portion is removed it may become revascularised by secondary, smaller feeding vessels.

The principle of total removal of the fistula would appear to apply to spinal angiomas, and as the precise site of the shunt cannot usually be identified at operation, the whole arterialised segment should be excised. This main mass may be quite extensive, and in this series has varied in length from 3 to $11\frac{1}{2}$ cm.

6 From the prognostic point of view, the influence on the angioma of temporary occlusion of its main arterial supply may be helpful. This was done in 13 of the 15 cases in this series which were approached intradurally, and in all but one there was some visible change in the malformation. These changes were sometimes delayed for up to 10 minutes, and ranged from:

(a) Marginal but detectable reduction in turgor and pulsation of the vessels, without colour change.

(b) More marked influence on turgor, with slight or no darkening in colour of the malformation.

(c) Pronounced reduction in pulsation, with marked colour change from arterial to venous.

In group (c) the changes appeared in less than 5 minutes (in one case in 15 seconds), and release of the clip usually reversed the colour changes in less than 30 seconds. There were 5 patients in this group and all had postoperative results which were among the best.

7 Postoperative selective angiography should be reregarded as essential. Although performed in only

2 patients in this series, it will be performed routinely in the future for the following reasons:

(a) To ensure that the angioma, with all its angiographically defined feeding vessels, has been removed.

(b) To see whether other feeding vessels have become visible and are filling small angiomatous remnants inadvertently left in the neighbourhood of the original lesion, or situated within the cord. This is of importance in assessing the future prognosis, and elucidating causes of later deterioration.

(c) When a portion of the angioma, perhaps within the cord, has been left behind, to demonstrate whether this still fills, possibly via vessels not previously demonstrated.

(d) To ascertain, in the occasional case in which serious deterioration has occurred postoperatively, whether there has been any interference with the main vessels feeding the anterior spinal artery.

The timing of this investigation is important, and if surgery has been uneventful it can perhaps be accomplished most suitably in the 3rd postoperative week. If a postoperative deterioration has occurred, however, it can be delayed for 4 to 6 weeks, or even longer. Late deterioration would seem to justify prompt reinvestigation by angiography.

Operative technique

EXPOSURE

1 In most cases removal of three laminae is the minimum required to provide adequate access and to ensure that the arterialised segment with its emergent veins is exposed, and this will need to be enlarged for more extensive angiomas. (A laminectomy of five vertebrae was the greatest required in this series.)

2 The theca is opened longitudinally, preferably with preservation of the arachnoid. This will show:

(a) In some cases the presence of an arachnoiditis.

(b) Whether the main feeding vessel is in the operative field.

(c) Whether the whole of the angioma is exposed; if it is not, further laminectomy can be done at this stage without the risk of excess blood entering the subarachnoid space.

3 The arachnoid is opened and adhesions are divided,

care being taken to avoid damaging any vessels at this stage.

Magnification in some form is very useful. A magnifying loupe is usually adequate but the operating microscope with its better light has many advantages, including the photographic recording of changes in pulsation and colour on temporary occlusion of feeders.

1 The main feeder is identified. If two have been shown at angiography but only one can be seen intradurally, extradural dissection is necessary to determine whether there has been an anastomosis extrathecally, and if not a further search, particularly among the nerve roots, should be made.

The main feeding vessel will usually be found entering the theca 2 to 3 mm away from the root sleeve; it may run upwards with the related root, but often takes a transverse or even obliquely downward course on to the spinal cord where it adopts its characteristic convoluted appearance, sometimes breaking up into several branches.

2 If the main feeder to the anterior spinal artery is known from the pre-operative angiographic studies to be in the vicinity, it must be defined and left undisturbed. It will be recognised by its longer, oblique but straight course, usually running with an anterior root on to the front of the cord.

3 A temporary clip is placed on the main feeding vessel to the angioma and the resulting changes are noted. If more than one feeder is present, this is done for each in turn, and then all are occluded together and the changes observed. If the requisite technical facilities are available, changes in pressure at various sites in the angioma may be recorded during this procedure. This may possibly be shown in the future to be helpful in determining the ultimate surgical outcome.

4 The feeding artery is occluded with clips, divided and followed on to the cord; the arterialised mass can usually be dissected off the cord substance for a good deal of its extent without damage to the pia. Sometimes the mass actually stands proud of the cord by a few mm. At intervals small vessels run into the cord substance. These presumably are important channels linking up with the parenchymatous venous circulation, and they are carefully coagulated with bipolar coagulation or clipped just short of the pia to avoid damage to posterior columns.

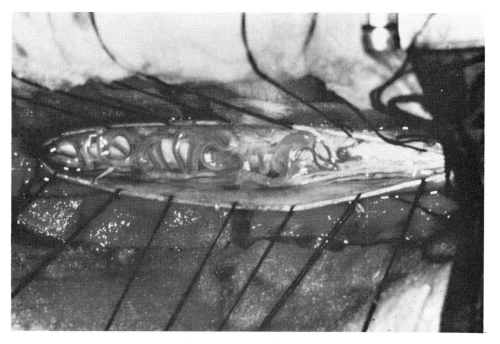

(a)

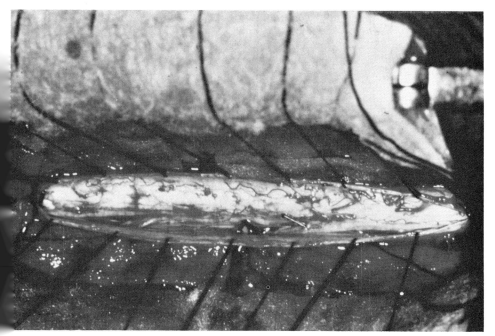

(b)

Figure 13.1. (a) Typical
operative appearance of a
lower thoracic angioma.

(b) Appearance following
removal of the malformation.
The clips are occluding the
main feeding vessel.

5 Vessels coming from the front of the cord to enter the angioma are divided, as are any recognisable branches from arteries supplying the anterior spinal once they have reached the back of the cord to enter the malformation.
6 The whole of the fistulous portion of the angioma is freed until the emergent veins are identified, and in a long anomaly this may need to be done in segments. The veins are clipped half a cm away from the angioma, and the collapsed mass is lifted away (Figure 13.1a, b).
7 At the conclusion, the pia should be intact except where any perforating vessels have been coagulated.
8 Where it is seen that part of the angioma lies within the substance of the cord, often producing a visible expansion of it, the vessels are sealed flush with the cord as they enter it, but otherwise are best left undisturbed. (This procedure was adopted in 3 patients, 2 of whom subsequently did well.)

CLOSURE

1 All blood is removed from the theca. The arachnoid layer is brought together over the cord where possible, and held in apposition with a few clips.
2 The dura is closed with a continuous suture to achieve a watertight closure; the muscles are brought together in layers with suction drainage to prevent a haematoma or the formation of a lake of cerebrospinal fluid.

Postoperative care

The usual routine care for patients subjected to spinal surgery is adopted, and most cases will require temporary catheterisation. Treatment with dexamethasone is started the day before operation and may be continued for several days, depending on progress. Cases showing neurological deterioration in the immediate postoperative period, or within the next few hours or days, may be helped by the use of mannitol in addition.

Appendix 1

In several chapters of this book, data were obtained by a personal analysis of the previously published literature. This was studied in detail, and only cases in which the malformation was considered to correspond with the type under discussion were used. The source of these cases is given below, but for brevity those published before 1940 are not included since their source is clearly indicated by Wyburn-Mason (1943) in his monograph. Some case-material had been published on more than one occasion, but details of these cases were included only once in the data which were analysed.

Aminoff and Logue, 1974a, b; Antoni, 1962; Arseni and Samitca, 1959; Bailey and Sperl, 1969; Bassett, Peet and Holt, 1949; Béraud and Meloche, 1965; Bergstrand, Höök and Lidvall, 1964; Brion, Netsky and Zimmerman, 1952; Buchanan and Walker, 1941; Cross, 1947; Den Hartog Jager, 1949; Djindjian, Houdart and Hurth, 1969; Djindjian, Hurth and Houdart, 1970; Doppman, Di Chiro and Ommaya, 1971; Echols and Holcombe, 1940–1; Epstein, Beller and Cohen, 1949; Fine, 1961; Gilbert, 1952; Girard and Garde, 1955; Gross and Ralston, 1959; Henson and Croft, 1956; Höök and Lidvall, 1958; Jackson and Hussey, 1967; Kaufman, Ommaya, Di Chiro and Doppman, 1970; Krayenbühl and Yaşargil, 1963; Krayenbühl, Yaşargil and McClintock, 1969; Kunc and Bret, 1969; Logue, Aminoff and Kendall, 1974; Lombardi and Migliavacca, 1959; Luessenhop and Dela Cruz, 1969; Matthews, 1959; Morris, 1960; Newman, 1959; Newquist and Mayfield, 1960; Nielsen, Marvin and Seletz, 1958; Odom, Woodhall and Margolis, 1957; Ommaya, Di Chiro and Doppman, 1969; Pouyanne, Bergouigan and Caillon, 1950; Ransome and Mekie, 1942; Roger, Paillas, Bonnal and Vigouroux, 1951; Schott, Cotte, Trillet and Bady, 1963; Scoville, 1948; Shephard, 1963, 1965; Stein, Ommaya, Doppman and Di Chiro, 1972; Strain, 1964; Szojchet, 1968; Teng and Papatheodorou, 1964; Teng and Shapiro, 1958; Therkelsen, 1958; Trupp and Sachs, 1948; Verbiest and Calliauw, 1960; Vraa-Jensen, 1949; Walton, 1953; Wirth, Post, Di Chiro, Doppman and Ommaya, 1970; Wyburn-Mason, 1943.

Appendix 2

In order to illustrate more fully the clinical and radiological features of spinal angiomas, the details of 16 cases are summarised below. All of these cases were operated upon by Professor V. Logue at the National Hospitals for Nervous Diseases in the last 10 years, and most of them exemplify the value of selective spinal angiography in delineating the malformation, and the benefit which follows surgical excision of its fistulous portion.

For brevity, irrelevant details and normal findings have been omitted, and comment has been restricted to a minimum. It should be emphasised, however, that symptoms commenced insidiously and progressed steadily in most cases, and were often aggravated by such factors as exercise or posture, while the signs were usually indicative of a lesion affecting several segments of the cord. It should also be noted that in several cases diagnosis was delayed because the underlying angioma was initially not recognised at myelography.

Case 1

Mr T.A., a 64-year-old solicitor, was admitted to hospital (A 50782) in 1969.

History

5 years previously he had had to rest in bed for several weeks because of low back pain. 2 or 3 years later he became unsteady on his feet, and after about a year he found he was impotent. 6 months later he developed hesitancy of micturition, followed by constipation and then by numbness and paraesthesiae in the right foot; this gradually spread up to the knee, the back of the thigh and the buttock, and then to the penis, scrotum and the back of the left thigh and buttock. He became more unsteady on his feet, his exercise tolerance diminished, and he found that he could not feel the passage of urine or faeces.

Examination

There was mild hypotonicity and weakness of both legs in a non-pyramidal distribution. The left knee jerk was brisker than the right, both ankle jerks were absent, and the plantar responses were extensor bilaterally. Pin-prick and light touch appreciation were impaired below the 3rd lumbar dermatome bilaterally, with relative sparing of the 4th and 5th sacral segments.

There was impairment of postural sense in the 5th digit of both feet, and the appreciation of vibration was impaired at the right ankle. The anal reflex was absent.

Investigations

Plain X-rays of the spine showed lumbarisation of the first part of the sacrum. The cerebrospinal fluid contained 1 cell per cu mm and a protein concentration of 85 mg per cent. Myelography initially showed no abnormality, but when more contrast medium was introduced subsequently, large tortuous vessels were outlined in the lower thoracic region, with smaller ones extending throughout the thoracic region on the posterior aspect of the cord. Selective spinal angiography showed an angioma which was fed by the right subcostal artery, while the artery of Adamkiewicz arose from the 2nd left lumbar artery; the arteriovenous shunt was located behind the cord at the level of the 11th thoracic vertebra, and tortuous draining veins extended to the upper thoracic region.

Surgery

After laminectomy of the 11th and 12th thoracic, and the 1st lumbar vertebrae, the exposed dura was incised to disclose the angioma. The prominent veins ascending and descending the cord contained bright red blood which darkened when the main vessel feeding the angioma was temporarily occluded. It was therefore divided just after its entry into the dura, and the convoluted coils of draining vessels were dissected off the cord, divided at the limits of the exposure, and removed. The dura, muscles and skin were then closed.

Subsequent course

He left hospital 4 weeks later, by which time sensory appreciation—particularly of cutaneous stimuli—had improved considerably, although there was little change in power. Further improvement occurred over the months, however, and when last reviewed, $4\frac{1}{4}$ years after operation, there was only slight residual leg weakness, sensory symptoms were confined to the right leg, and he was able to walk as far as he wished without difficulty; nevertheless, his mild disturbance of micturition and defaecation persisted, and he remained impotent.

Comment

The initial myelographic studies failed to reveal any significant abnormality in spite of screening in both prone and supine positions, and it was only when more contrast material was introduced (to make a total of 21 cc in all) that the angioma was found. His previously progressive downhill course was arrested by surgical excision of the fistulous portion of the malformation, and there has been a considerable return of functional capacity since operation.

Case 2

Mr C.B., a 47-year-old sales manager, was admitted (A 48639) in 1969.

History

He complained of increasing weakness in the legs, initially related to exercise, for $2\frac{1}{2}$ years. His exercise tolerance gradually diminished, he took to walking with sticks, and 6 months before admission he became chairbound. His condition continued to deteriorate, and eventually he was unable even to move his legs in bed. 1 year before admission he developed hesitancy of micturition and intermittent retention of urine, and became constipated. Over the following months he developed a dull ache in the back, numbness in the left buttock, painful paraesthesiae in the legs, faecal incontinence, and persistent urinary retention which necessitated catheterisation. He was investigated elsewhere about a year after the onset of symptoms, but the angioma was not recognised at myelography.

Examination

The legs were wasted and hypotonic, and power in them was so reduced that he was virtually paraplegic. The abdominal reflexes were absent as were the tendon reflexes in the legs, and both plantar responses were extensor. All modalities of cutaneous sensation were impaired below the 2nd lumbar dermatomes except in a few scattered patches, postural sense was impaired below the knees, and vibration could not be felt below the costal margin. The anal sphincter was lax and he had an indwelling bladder catheter. A decubitus ulcer was present over the sacrum.

Investigations

Review of the films of his previous myelogram showed that tortuous vessels were abnormally prominent in the upper thoracic region. Selective spinal angiography demonstrated an angioma supplied only by the 8th right intercostal artery, while the artery of Adamkiewicz arose from the 10th right intercostal; the arterial component of the malformation was situated posteriorly at the level of the 7th and 8th thoracic vertebrae, and extensive, tortuous, draining veins were seen posteriorly in the spinal canal between the 4th and 9th thoracic vertebrae.

Surgery

After laminectomy of the 7th, 8th and 9th thoracic vertebrae, the dura and arachnoid were opened to expose the angioma. Its feeding artery was easily identified, but temporary occlusion of this vessel caused little visible change in the malformation. The artery broke into several branches which supplied a tangle of arterialised veins, but it was not possible to recognise the precise site of the arteriovenous shunt. The exposed vessels were divided at the limits of the exposure, and the angioma was removed. The subjacent cord was undisturbed, and did not look degenerate or oedematous. The wound was then closed in layers.

Subsequent course

As soon as he recovered consciousness, it was evident that the power in his legs had already improved, and by the time he left hospital, 6 weeks later, he could stand between parallel bars. His improvement continued, and when last reviewed $4\frac{1}{2}$ years later, he was able to walk about 100 yards with 2 sticks; his sensory symptoms had improved but remained troublesome, and he complained of constipation and occasional urinary incontinence.

Comment

There was a delay in establishing the diagnosis because the vascular shadows seen at myelography were originally considered to be within normal limits. He accordingly became severely disabled before the diagnosis was made, but his motor, sensory and sphincter disturbances improved after operation and he recovered a useful degree of function in the legs.

Case 3

Mr W.B., a 63-year-old photographer, was admitted to hospital (A 26156) in 1968.

History

5 years previously he had developed constipation, and this was followed by increasing numbness, weakness and stiffness in the legs, aggravated by exercise. He then developed urgency and occasional hesitancy of micturition and became impotent. In 1964, and again in 1965, myelography showed a partial obstruction between the 10th and 11th thoracic vertebrae suggestive of a prolapsed disc, and was followed by a deterioration in his condition; he was unable to walk without a stick after the first myelogram, and had transient urinary retention after the second. Neurosurgical exploration was deferred, and his condition continued to deteriorate. He developed further episodes of urinary retention, and in 1966 and 1967 he had a transurethral resection of the prostate gland on three separate occasions; after the last, which was done under spinal anaesthesia, his legs became weaker and he lost all control of micturition. He was able to walk about 50 yards with 2 sticks or crutches until 5 weeks prior to admission, however, when the weakness increased following physiotherapy at home and he was unable to stand without assistance.

Examination

He had a dorsal kyphosis. There was weakness of the lower abdominal muscles, and the cutaneous reflexes could not be elicited below the umbilicus. In the legs, tone was increased proximally but reduced distally, and there was generalised weakness. The knee jerks were pathologically brisk, the ankle jerks were absent, and the plantar responses were unobtainable. All modalities of cutaneous sensation were impaired up to the 11th thoracic dermatome bilaterally, postural sense was severely impaired in both legs, and vibration could not be felt below the costal margin. The anal sphincter was lax, the anal reflex was absent, and he was wearing a urinary incontinence appliance. He could not stand without assistance.

Investigations

Review of the myelogram performed in 1965 suggested that there were some abnormally prominent vascular impressions in the thoracic region. An aortogram showed hypertrophy of a radicular artery in the lower thoracic region, but selective injection of the intercostal arteries could not be performed.

Surgery

Laminectomy of the 9th, 10th, 11th and 12th thoracic vertebrae revealed an opaque dura which was incised. There was evidence of gross arachnoiditis, and enmeshed in the thickened arachnoid was a tightly coiled angioma. A large, tortuous vessel ran on the dorsum of the cord, and as it descended it was joined by a small artery, and then by a large vein and at least 2 larger arteries running with the 11th left nerve root; in the caudal part of the exposure it suddenly narrowed into a small arterial vessel which gradually made its way to the anterior aspect of the cord. These vessels were divided and dissected off the cord which looked grey and degenerate posteriorly. Exploration of its anterior aspect revealed no extension of the angioma, and the wound was therefore closed.

Subsequent course

He showed little change in his condition in the immediate postoperative period, but over the months he regained some power and sensation in the legs. When last reviewed, $5\frac{1}{2}$ years after operation, he was able to walk about $\frac{1}{8}$th of a mile with 2 sticks and his sensory symptoms were less intrusive. He remained impotent and incontinent of urine, however, and although his bowels were opened regularly, there was very occasional faecal soiling.

Comment

Diagnosis was delayed because the myelographic appearances were abnormal but atypical. He nevertheless showed a gratifying recovery of some useful function in the legs after operation.

Case 4

Mr S.C., a 64-year-old engineer, was readmitted to hospital (A 42041) in 1972.

History

He was first admitted in 1968 with an 18-month history of numbness in the legs which had commenced insidiously and gradually extended to the waist. He had been impotent and had hesitancy of micturition for about a year, and his legs had felt stiff and heavy for several weeks prior to admission. Examination revealed a mild spastic paraparesis with impairment of cutaneous sensation below the 2nd thoracic dermatomes and of deep sensibility in the legs. Myelography showed irregular, tortuous shadows from the cervical to the lumbar region; there was no obstruction in the subarachnoid space and the cord was not expanded. A diagnosis of spinal angioma was made and he was followed up as an outpatient.

Over the following 3½ years weakness and stiffness of the legs—enhanced by exercise, straining at stool or hot baths—gradually increased in severity until eventually he could only walk with the support of 2 sticks, and the numbness also became more intense. He became increasingly constipated, was occasionally incontinent of faeces, developed frequency of micturition with urgency and occasional incontinence, and began to experience frequent flexor spasms in the legs.

Examination

There was spasticity and marked pyramidal weakness of both legs, with brisk tendon reflexes but flexor plantar responses. The abdominal reflexes were absent. Pinprick appreciation was impaired below the 6th, and lost below the 11th thoracic segments, and touch was impaired below the 12th; vibration could not be felt below the iliac crests, and there was gross postural loss in the legs.

Investigations

Selective spinal angiography demonstrated an angioma situated posteriorly at the level of the 6th and 7th thoracic vertebrae. It was fed by the 7th and 8th right intercostal arteries, and the major source of supply to the anterior spinal artery in this region was the 9th left intercostal.

Surgery

The dura was exposed by laminectomy of the 5th, 6th, 7th and 8th thoracic vertebrae, and on opening it the angioma was immediately visible. There were a number of small, tortuous vessels rostrally and a single, larger vein caudally. The actual shunt seemed to be in the centre of the field and was supplied by two arteries which joined at the level of the 7th nerve root; from their confluence two further vessels emerged, the larger of which supplied the angioma directly while the other ran along the posterior root to enter the malformation 2 cm more rostrally. Temporary clipping of the lower artery led to a slow darkening in colour of the vein situated inferiorly, but when the second feeder was clipped there was a more rapid darkening of all the anomalous vessels. The feeding arteries and large draining vein were divided and the angioma was dissected off the cord; in the upper half of the exposure, small veins running round the side of the cord from the main mass of vessels were coagulated, and two vessels which extended more rostrally along the dorsum of the cord were divided. The angioma was then removed and the wound was closed.

Subsequent course

His neurological deficit was initially increased, but he gradually became more mobile and within a month he could get about the ward with 2 sticks. When seen last 2 years later, he had regained considerable power in the legs but nevertheless still required 2 sticks to get about with facility. His sensory symptoms and signs were less conspicuous, but he remained impotent and constipated, with occasional faecal incontinence. The control of micturition also remained disturbed, and he emptied his bladder by manual compression every 2 hours because he was unable to appreciate when it was full.

Comment

This case illustrates the extensive abnormalities which are sometimes found at myelography and the value of selective spinal angiography in permitting the most appropriate site for laminectomy to be recognised. It also emphasises the importance of early surgical treatment, because this patient showed little functional recovery after operation, although his previously progressive downhill course was arrested.

Case 5

Mr J.B., a 63-year-old retired insurance salesman, was readmitted (67589) in 1972.

History

He was first admitted in 1969 with a 3 year history of increasing weakness in the legs which originally was related to exercise, relieved by a brief rest and accompanied by an ache in the knees. For 2 years he had also had paraesthesiae in the legs and fingers, and for 1 year had experienced urgency and hesitancy of micturition. Examination revealed a mild spastic paraparesis with brisk reflexes and bilateral extensor plantar responses, but no sensory signs. Myelography showed serpiginous defects both anterior and posterior to the cord from the mid-cervical to lower lumbar region, suggestive of an angioma. He was able to get about with a stick, and in view of his relatively mild disability surgery was deferred.

His weakness gradually increased over the months. Early in 1971 it began to progress more rapidly soon after an episode of back pain which occurred while he was bending forward, and he started to use 2 sticks for walking; by the end of that year he was virtually confined to bed. Over that time he also developed impotence, constipation, occasional faecal incontinence, numbness in the legs, recurrent retention of urine and occasional urinary incontinence. He was therefore readmitted for further assessment.

Examination

The lower abdominal muscles were weak and there was a severe spastic paraparesis. The abdominal reflexes were absent, all the tendon reflexes were pathologically brisk, and both plantar responses were equivocal. Pin-prick and, to a lesser extent, light touch appreciation were impaired below the 10th thoracic dermatomes, postural sense was impaired in both legs, and vibration could not be felt below the iliac crests.

Investigations

Selective spinal angiography demonstrated that the angioma, which was situated postero-laterally at the 6th thoracic vertebral level, was fed by the 6th right intercostal artery, while the artery of Adamkiewicz was supplied by the 9th left intercostal. The procedure was followed by a transient increase in his motor and sensory symptoms, and he developed urinary retention which necessitated catheterisation.

Operation

After laminenctomy of the 5th, 6th and 7th thoracic vertebrae, the dura was incised to expose the angioma which completely covered the back of the cord and consisted of tight coils of pulsating anomalous vessels. The feeding artery divided into an ascending and descending branch which ramified over the cord surface; its temporary occlusion caused little colour change in the anomalous vessels, but their pulsation became less prominent. The main feeding vessel was divided, and the coiled vessels were dissected off the cord for about $2\frac{1}{2}$ inches and then divided. The remaining vessels, which extended rostrally and caudally from the excised region, were the colour of normal veins, indicating that the fistulous portion of the angioma had been removed. The dura, muscles and skin were then closed in layers.

Subsequent course

Weakness in the legs became more marked in the immediate postoperative period, but over the weeks it improved steadily, as did his sensory symptoms. He was last reviewed 2 years later when he was able to get about with 2 sticks, but his disturbance of micturition and defaecation remained as severe as it was pre-operatively.

Comment

Treatment was delayed in this case because the patient's incapacity was relatively mild when the diagnosis was first made. Progression continued inexorably, however, and his resulting disability was only improved in part by excision of the fistula. The value of selective spinal angiography in localising the site of the shunt is well exemplified, for the findings at myelography would certainly not have permitted the accurate siting of a laminectomy.

Case 6

Mr E.S., a 53-year-old engineer, was admitted (A 35108) in 1967.

History

In 1964 he sustained minor injuries in a road traffic accident, and a few months later he developed increasing dysaesthesiae in the buttocks and back of both legs, which occurred when he was sitting and were relieved by standing. About a year later he developed hesitancy of micturition and constipation, with an accompanying impairment of rectal sensation, while the dysaesthesiae gradually spread further in the legs. A few months after this, he noticed weakness of the legs which was aggravated by sitting, so that his right leg would fall off the accelerator pedal if he drove for more than 40 miles in his car. He was investigated elsewhere by myelography, but the presence of an angioma was not recognised. The weakness in the legs gradually became more severe, but fluctuated in severity so that his exercise tolerance varied between 50 and 150 yards; it was always aggravated by bending forward. In the few months before referral to the National Hospital, he also developed flexor spasms of both legs, and his hesitancy of micturition became more severe.

Examination

There was wasting of the buttocks and left calf, and mild generalised weakness in the legs. The abdominal reflexes were absent in the lower quadrants, the tendon reflexes were depressed in the left leg, and the plantar responses were both extensor. The anus was patulous and the anal reflex was diminished. There was hyperalgesia and impairment of light touch appreciation in the sacral segments, and vibration was not felt at the ankles.

Investigations

The cerebrospinal fluid contained 1 lymphocyte per cu mm and a protein concentration of 100 mg per cent. Myelography showed serpiginous shadows both posterior and anterior to the cord between the 6th cervical and 2nd lumbar vertebrae. Aortography failed to outline the malformation.

Surgery

The dura was opened after laminectomy of the 10th, 11th and 12th thoracic, and 1st lumbar vertebrae. A large tortuous angioma was exposed on the dorsal surface of the cord, which looked slightly swollen. It comprised two large tortuous channels which contained arterial blood flowing in a rostral direction. Neither the artery of Adamkiewicz nor an artery feeding the angioma could be identified with certainty, but at least two vessels emerged from the surface of the cord to join the anomalous channels on the dorsum of the cord. The angiomatous vessels were divided, dissected off the cord and removed, and the wound was then closed in layers.

Subsequent course

His postoperative course was uncomplicated and over the weeks his motor and sensory symptoms improved. He was last reviewed 7 years after operation, when his exercise tolerance was unrestricted and he was able to drive his car for as long as he wished without difficulty. His dysasethesiae had cleared, and the control of micturition and defaecation was virtually normal.

Comment

Selective spinal angiography was not performed and it was therefore more difficult to identify any arteries feeding the malformation and localise the site of the shunt at operation. Since the excised vessels had contained arterial blood, however, they were presumably closely related to the shunt itself. The presence of local cord swelling, and of vessels emerging from the cord to connect with the angiomatous vessels suggests that there was an intramedullary component of the malformation, but he made a good functional recovery after operation and has remained well for 7 years.

Case 7

Mr J.deQ., a 55-year-old landscape gardener, was admitted (A 55886) in 1970.

History

In 1941 he developed severe weakness and numbness in the legs, and was admitted to hospital elsewhere; he eventually made a good recovery, but no diagnosis was made. He remained well until 1969, when he developed paraesthesiae which commenced in the toes and gradually ascended to the knees, while sensation became increasingly impaired below the waist. Two months after their onset he developed slowly progressive weakness of the legs, and his exercise tolerance eventually diminished to 25 yards. Over the months he also became aware of urgency and hesitancy of micturition, an inability to appreciate when the bladder was full, impotence, constipation and mild low back pain.

Examination

There was slight weakness of the lower abdominal muscles and general weakness of both legs, more marked on the right. The abdominal reflexes were absent, the left knee jerk was pathologically brisk, the right ankle jerk was depressed and the plantar responses were both extensor. The appreciation of pin-prick and, to a lesser extent, light touch was impaired below the 8th thoracic dermatomes, vibration appreciation was mildly impaired in both legs, and postural sense was slightly disturbed in the toes.

Investigations

The cerebrospinal fluid contained no cells and a protein concentration of 40 mg per cent. Myelography showed serpiginous filling defects on both anterior and posterior aspects of the cord throughout the thoracic region, and there was some swelling of the cord at the level of the 11th thoracic vertebra. Selective spinal angiography demonstrated that the angioma was situated posteriorly at the 4th thoracic vertebral level; its sole feeder was the 4th right intercostal artery, and it drained both rostrally and caudally, while the artery of Adamkiewicz arose from the 8th right intercostal. Following the procedure the weakness in his legs became more severe for a few days.

Surgery

After laminectomy of the 2nd, 3rd and 4th thoracic vertebrae, the dura was opened to expose the angioma. A large artery entered with the 4th right nerve root, ran on to the back of the cord, and made several loops as it ascended for about 3 cm to join with two vessels of similar size; one of these ascended while the other descended, and their point of confluence seemed to be the site of the shunt. When the main feeding artery was temporarily occluded, the other two vessels darkened and became less turgid over 1–2 minutes. All three vessels were therefore divided and dissected off the cord, and the wound was closed in layers.

Subsequent course

His postoperative course was uneventful and his motor and sensory deficit gradually improved. When last seen as an outpatient, 2 years after operation, his exercise tolerance was unrestricted and sensation in the left leg was virtually normal. However, he continued to have painful paraesthesiae and a sensory deficit in the right leg, the control of micturition and defaecation remained impaired, and he was still impotent.

Comment

The value of selective spinal angiography in localising the site of the fistula and origin of its feeding artery is well exemplified by this case. The patient's somatic symptoms and signs improved considerably after operation, in contrast to his disturbance of sphincter and sexual function.

Case 8

Mr C.C., a 60-year-old inspector of livestock, was admitted to hospital (A 56203) in 1970.

History

For 2–3 years he had experienced intermittent, painful cramps in the thighs and legs when sitting down, and some months after their onset, he began to catch his left foot while walking. His symptoms gradually progressed in severity, his legs became increasingly weak and thin, and 6 months before admission he started to use a stick for walking. At about this time, he also developed constipation and hesitancy of micturition. There was a long past history of ankylosing spondylitis.

Examination

The lower abdominal muscles were weak, but the cutaneous abdominal reflexes were preserved. There was wasting of the buttocks and left thigh, and fasciculation over both thighs. Tone was probably normal, but there was generalised weakness in both legs, especially the left. The ankle jerks were depressed and both plantar responses were equivocal. Pin-prick appreciation was impaired below the 12th left thoracic dermatome, with some sacral sparing, but there was hyperpathia bilaterally in the 12th thoracic and 1st lumbar dermatomes. Vibration appreciation was impaired below the left knee and at the right ankle. Light touch and joint position sense were normal. His gait was unsteady and he dragged his left leg.

Plain X-rays of the spine showed a slight scoliosis concave to the left, and in the lumbar region there was calcification of the longitudinal ligament and ankylosis of the sacro-iliac joint. The cerebrospinal fluid contained 1 lymphocyte per cu mm and a protein concentration of 60 mg per cent. Myelography showed serpiginous filling defects in the lower thoracic region without evidence of obstruction; at least some of these defects were anterior to the cord. Selective spinal angiography showed an angioma with the shunt situated posteriorly at the level of the 10th thoracic vertebra; it was fed by a solitary vessel ascending from the left subcostal artery, while the artery of Adamkiewicz arose from the 10th left intercostal. The procedure was followed by transient urinary retention which necessitated catheterisation.

Surgery

Laminectomy was performed, the dura incised, and the angioma exposed. It was situated both anterior and posterior to the cord; its feeding artery entered with the left 12th thoracic root, curled up the back of the cord, and at the level of the 10th thoracic vertebra divided into a branch passing anteriorly and a second branch which supplied a collection of abnormal vessels on the posterior surface of the cord. This knot of vessels was also fed by small arterial branches which came round the side of the cord from its anterior aspect. The artery of Adamkiewicz was identified, and was left undisturbed. Temporary occlusion of the vessel feeding the angioma caused a reduction of tension in the malformation. The artery was divided just within the dura and at its bifurcation, and removed. The abnormal collection of vessels on the dorsum of the cord was dissected free, and small arterial branches to it from the front of the cord were coagulated; the mass of vessels was divided caudally and removed just before it broke up into a number of fine branches which intermingled with the descending nerve roots. The wound was then closed in layers.

Subsequent course

His postoperative course was uneventful and his condition improved with time. Power in the legs increased so that he could get about without any support, and the control of micturition became virtually normal. When last reviewed $2\frac{1}{2}$ years after operation, however, he was still complaining of intermittent pain in the legs.

Comment

This case clearly demonstrates the value of selective spinal angiography, which permitted the topography of the malformation and the source of its feeding artery and the artery of Adamkiewicz to be identified pre-operatively. A worthwhile degree of functional recovery followed surgery, but an anterior extension of the angioma was left *in situ* and may lead to further symptoms if part of its blood supply was left intact. The value of postoperative angiography in such circumstances is readily apparent.

Case 9

Mr W.W., a 50-year-old industrial radiologist, was admitted (A 67666) in 1972.

History

A few days after a fall in 1969, he developed pain in the back and leg, and numbness of the left little toe. He was treated elsewhere by bilateral leg traction, but after 10 days he became aware of leg weakness and unsteadiness while walking. The pain persisted and was aggravated by walking, while his weakness slowly advanced so that within a year he was finding it difficult to rise from a chair. In 1971 he began to have nocturnal flexor spasms. He then developed transient episodes of numbness in the right leg, precipitated by maintaining his legs in one position for any length of time. His weakness continued to increase, and 8 months before admission he had a myelogram elsewhere without the angioma being recognised; he was manipulated under anaesthesia and the following day found that the left leg was numb. A diagnosis of multiple sclerosis was eventually made and a course of ACTH prescribed; 4 hours after the first injection, however, there was a transient but severe exacerbation of the weakness and numbness in his legs, and treatment was discontinued when this recurred after a second injection. His symptoms continued to progress, and by the time of his referral to the National Hospital he was sometimes too weak to walk at all and both his legs were numb. When admitted, he also complained of episodic low back pain radiating to the right leg, occasional urinary incontinence and constipation.

Examination

The buttocks were wasted, and there was spasticity and profound global weakness of the legs with absent or diminished tendon reflexes and extensor plantar responses. The abdominal reflexes were absent below the level of the umbilicus. Temperature and pin-prick appreciation were impaired in both legs, with an ill-defined level at the 10th thoracic dermatome, but light touch appreciation was impaired only over the feet. The appreciation of vibration was impaired below the iliac crests and postural sense was disturbed at the ankles and knees, but preserved in the toes.

Investigations

The contrast material had been allowed to remain in the subarachnoid space after his previous myelogram, and rescreening revealed serpiginous defects suggestive of an angioma in the lower thoracic region. Spinal angiography showed that the angioma was supplied only by a hypertrophied branch of the 11th left intercostal artery, while the artery of Adamkiewicz arose from the 10th left intercostal; the shunt was on the left side of the cord at the 10th thoracic vertebral level, and its venous drainage was extensive in both rostral and caudal directions.

Surgery

The angioma was exposed by laminectomy of the 9th, 10th and 11th thoracic vertebrae and incision of the subjacent dura. Its feeding artery was easily identified; it ascended for about 3 cm on to the back of the cord, and gave off three apparently venous channels, one ascending the cord, another descending, and the third running between the left 10th and 11th nerve roots. There was considerable arachnoiditis, and the arachnoid overlying the lesion was carefully removed. The feeding artery was clipped, and within 15 seconds all the exposed vessels became progressively darker; on releasing the clip they rapidly flushed with bright red blood. The entering artery and its three branches were divided, dissected off the cord and removed. The wound was then closed in layers.

Subsequent course

His condition showed little change immediately after operation, but 4 days later his paresis became almost complete. This was attributed to cord ischaemia and oedema, and he was treated with a brief course of oral steroids. He began to improve after a few days and within a month his power was better than it had been pre-operatively. After 2 months he could walk with crutches, and 2 months later he could walk unsupported for short distances. When last seen, 1 year after operation, he had recovered considerable power in the legs and could walk for about 3 miles with 2 sticks or for short distances without any support; sensory symptoms and signs were less conspicuous and micturition was normal, but he remained with mild constipation and had some urgency of defaecation.

Comment

The clinical course in this patient was one of steady progression, but a spurious impression of episodic progression resulted from the aggravation of symptoms which occurred in relation to posture, manipulation, and ACTH administration. A worthwhile degree of functional recovery followed surgery.

Case 10

Mrs U.P., a 33-year-old housewife, was admitted to hospital (A 59239) in 1971.

History

At the age of 6 years she developed weakness in the legs which made it difficult for her to climb stairs, but this gradually settled. She was otherwise well until she was 23 years old when, during her first pregnancy, she developed left-sided sciatica which recurred in both of her subsequent pregnancies and on other occasions over the following years. The pain was often brought on by bending forward or turning in bed, and was relieved by rest. Five months before admission she developed a dull pain in the back, radiating to the groins, thighs, vagina and rectum, and at about this time she became aware of a mild but persistent weakness in the legs. Two weeks before admission, while bending down, she developed sudden weakness of both legs and numbness over the buttocks, and subsequently found that she was unable to empty her bladder or bowels. Although the weakness and numbness improved in part over a few days, her control of micturition and defaecation remained severely impaired; she was accordingly referred to the National Hospital and admitted forthwith.

Examination

There was wasting of the left buttock, increased tone and variable weakness of both legs, and a patchy impairment of pin-prick and temperature appreciation in the sacral dermatomes, with preservation of light touch appreciation. The abdominal reflexes were absent, the tendon reflexes in the legs were brisk, and the right plantar response was flexor while the left was unobtainable. The anus was patulous, the anal reflex was absent, and a bladder catheter was *in situ*. There was considerable fluctuation in the severity of her signs over relatively short intervals; at times she was hardly able to maintain the position of her legs against gravity, while on other occasions she could walk but dragged her right leg.

Investigations

Plain X-rays of the spine showed a slight scoliosis to the left in the lower thoracic region. The cerebrospinal fluid contained 1 lymphocyte per cu mm and a protein concentration of 120 mg per cent. Myelography showed enlargement of the conus at the level of the first lumbar vertebra and constant serpiginous defects in the lumbar subarachnoid space. Spinal angiography showed an angioma supplied by the 2nd right lumbar and 10th left intercostal arteries, while the artery of Adamkiewicz arose from the left subcostal artery and did not supply the malformation; the shunt was situated posteriorly at the level of the 1st lumbar vertebra and drained to veins situated both anterior and posterior to the cord, particularly in a rostral direction.

Surgery

Laminectomy of the 12th thoracic and 1st lumbar vertebrae was performed. The dura was not tense, and on opening it a pulsating mass of convoluted vessels was exposed. The angioma was about $2\frac{1}{2}$ cm in vertical extent, 2 cm in transverse diameter, and was elevated from the back of the cord by about 6 mm. A large vein ascended from it on the dorsum of the cord, and a further trunk descended over the nerve roots, where a number of fine arteries and veins were also found. The main feeding trunk from the 2nd right lumbar artery could not be identified, but two large vessels which probably derived from it came round from the front of the cord and joined the upper part of the malformation. When these were temporarily occluded there was a reduction in tension of the angiomatous mass but it continued to pulsate. They were divided and dissected off the cord, as was the ascending venous trunk. The rest of the angioma was followed caudally where a number of small arteries were found to enter it from the cord itself. The dissection was continued, and a large vessel, occluded by recent blood clot, was seen to run from the inferior aspect of the angioma into the cauda equina. As the angioma was freed, the subjacent cord was seen to be swollen and a number of tough venous channels were seen to connect the extramedullary lesion with the cord. These vessels were divided, the angioma was removed, all bleeding was arrested and the wound was closed in layers.

Subsequent course

Her condition gradually improved and within 2 months she was able to walk without difficulty for as far as she wished. When last seen 3 years later her exercise tolerance was unrestricted and the control of micturition was virtually normal, but she remained with mild constipation and impaired genital sensation.

Comment

This patient's presenting symptoms were of acute onset and may well have related to intravascular thrombosis, for a large vessel was found at operation to be occluded by recent blood clot. There was considerable recovery of function after surgery; she may well have had an intramedullary extension of the angioma, however, and this may lead to further symptoms if part of its blood supply remains intact.

Case 11

Mr A.D., a 58-year-old salesman, was admitted (A 53748) in 1970.

History

About a year before admission he first noticed numbness in the sole of the right foot, and shortly afterwards his legs began to feel heavy toward the end of the day and he became constipated. Weakness of the legs gradually progressed and they began to waste. Three months after the onset of symptoms he developed shooting pains in the legs and soon afterwards a loss of feeling in the bladder and rectum, and occasional urinary incontinence. Myelography was performed elsewhere at this time, but the angioma was not recognised. Over the following months walking became progressively more difficult and he developed persistent numbness in the legs. His disturbance of micturition also increased to retention and overflow incontinence which necessitated catheterisation, and he developed impotence and occasional faecal incontinence. He was admitted elsewhere and transferred to the National Hospital after investigations had revealed the presence of an angioma.

Examination

There was marked wasting in both legs, affecting particularly the glutei and hamstrings. There was generalised weakness in the legs, the ankle jerks were absent and the plantar responses were equivocal. A band of hypalgesia was present in both groins, and there was dense hypalgesia below the knees, spreading to the saddle area in which there was complete analgesia. Vibration was not felt below the iliac crests. The anal reflex was absent and a bladder catheter was *in situ*. He was able to walk a few paces with a stick.

Investigation

These were performed elsewhere. Rescreening of the contrast material from his previous myelogram showed abnormally prominent vessels in the lower thoracic region. Angiography demonstrated an angioma situated posteriorly at the level of the 9th and 10th thoracic vertebrae; it was supplied by the 9th right intercostal artery, while the artery of Adamkiewicz arose from the 11th right intercostal.

Operation

After laminectomy of the 9th, 10th and 11th thoracic vertebrae, the dura was opened and a large, pulsating vessel was seen to enter with the 9th right nerve root and make a tortuous descent on the posterior surface of the cord for about 4 cm before straightening out and continuing toward the conus. One or two small vessels ran from it into the cord. Temporary occlusion of its rostral end caused only slight reduction in pulsation. The entering artery was divided and dissected off the cord as far as the lower limit of the exposure where it was divided again and removed. The wound was then closed in layers.

Subsequent course

Within a few days it became clear that there was marked improvement in power and sensation in both legs. When last seen 4 years later, he remained incontinent of urine and was constipated, but he was able to walk without a stick although his exercise tolerance was restricted.

Comment

This patient's rapidly progressive downhill course was arrested by surgery. His somatic symptoms improved considerably, but his sphincter disturbance remained severe.

Case 12

Mrs E.H., a 73-year-old housewife, was admitted to hospital (A 70782) in 1973.

History

She had had weakness in the legs for 18 months; this began insidiously and progressed steadily until she was unable to walk at all. Over this time she had also developed paraesthesiae and numbness in the legs, occasional low back pain, and a disturbance of micturition characterised initially by urgency and subsequently by urinary retention with overflow incontinence which necessitated catheterisation.

Examination

The buttocks, thighs and calves were wasted. There was an increase in tone and generalised weakness in both legs. The lower abdominal reflexes were absent, both ankle jerks were pathologically brisk, and the plantar responses were extensor bilaterally. All modalities of cutaneous sensation were impaired below the right 9th and left 11th thoracic dermatomes, postural sense was impaired in the toes of both feet, and vibration could not be felt below the iliac crests. A bladder catheter was *in situ*.

Investigations

The cerebrospinal fluid contained 1 white cell per cu mm and a protein concentration of 75 mg per cent. Myelography showed a number of vermiform defects over the surface of the cord, suggestive of an extensive angioma in the lower thoracic region. Selective spinal angiography showed the malformation to lie on the right postero-lateral aspect of the cord at the level of the 9th thoracic vertebra; it was fed from the 8th and 9th right intercostal arteries, while the major supply to the anterior spinal artery was from the 7th left intercostal.

Surgery

An attempt was made to occlude the vessels feeding the angioma by embolism with gel-foam, but angiographic re-examination 24 days later showed that both feeders were still patent. Accordingly, laminectomy of the 7th, 8th and 9th thoracic vertebrae was performed and the dura incised to expose the angioma. It consisted of a single, coiled vessel which gave off several branches inferiorly where there were a number of fine, twisted vessels running in the arachnoid and along the nerve roots. The artery of Adamkiewicz was identified, but only a single feeding vessel to the malformation could be found although two had been demonstrated at angiography. The feeder branched into two vessels which passed to the dorsum of the cord, one ascending as a single channel while the other turned downward and divided into two intertwining vessels which disappeared beyond the limits of the exposure. Temporary occlusion of the feeding vessel caused only a slight change in colour and reduction in tension of the angioma. The main vessel and its branches were dissected off the cord, divided and removed, and the wound was closed in layers.

Subsequent course

There was no significant change in her symptoms and signs in the weeks following operation. Some improvement in power occurred subsequently, but 9 months after operation she was able to get about only with the support of a frame and help of a nurse. Her disturbance of micturition had improved sufficiently to permit removal of her catheter, but she was occasionally incontinent of urine.

Comment

Although an attempt to occlude the blood supply to the angioma by embolisation was unsuccessful in this case, others have reported some success with the procedure. The patient's rapidly progressive downhill course was arrested by excision of the fistula but she remained severely disabled. One of the two segmental feeding vessels seen at angiography was not identified at operation, possibly because it was not looked for in the extra-dural tissues (in contrast to Case 13); this indicates the importance of removing the fistulous portion of the malformation in addition to dividing any feeding arteries which can be recognised.

Case 13

Mr T.W., a 51-year-old train driver, was admitted (76499) in 1973.

History

Two months before admission he developed episodic pain in the right leg which was brought on by exercise and relieved by rest. One week later both legs became swollen and he was admitted to his local hospital. Over the next few days he developed rapidly progressive weakness in the legs, urinary retention and faecal incontinence. His cerebrospinal fluid was examined and found to contain 28 white cells per cu mm (70 per cent polymorphs) and a protein concentration of 60 mg per cent. Myelography initially revealed no abnormality, but after rescreening a few days later the presence of an angioma was suspected. He remained severely disabled, unable to walk without support, although slight improvement occurred over the next few weeks. He was then transferred to Maida Vale Hospital.

Examination

There was weakness of the lower abdominal muscles, with absent cutaneous reflexes on the right side. He had a severe flaccid paraparesis with absent tendon reflexes and bilateral extensor plantar responses. Pin-prick and, to a lesser extent, light touch appreciation were impaired below the 2nd right lumbar and 12th left thoracic dermatomes, postural sense was grossly impaired proximally in both legs, and the appreciation of vibration was impaired below the iliac crests. A bladder catheter was *in situ.*

Investigations

Selective spinal angiography showed a malformation which was situated on the right postero-lateral aspect of the cord at the level of the 9th thoracic vertebra. It was fed by the 9th and a descending branch of the 8th right intercostal arteries, while the artery of Adamkiewicz arose from the 10th left intercostal.

Operation

After laminectomy of the 7th, 8th, 9th and part of the 10th thoracic vertebrae the dura was excised to expose the angioma. Just below the 9th right thoracic root, a large vessel entered and immediately broke up into three vessels which ramified on the back of the cord; one ascended to a group of anomalous vessels, the second ran directly across the cord to another knot of vessels, while the third ran down as a long, tortuous channel. The feeder from the 8th intercostal artery could not be identified within the dura. Temporary clipping of the other feeder led to a darkening in colour of the anomalous vessels over about 5 minutes, but when the clip was removed they reverted to their original reddish hue within 15 seconds. The entering artery and its three main branches were divided and dissected off the cord, as were the two groups of vessels which they joined. The right extradural tissues were then exposed and a knot of vessels was found just below the 9th nerve root, with a small arterial channel running down to it from the artery accompanying the 8th root. This was left undisturbed and the wound was closed in layers.

Subsequent course

His condition was initially unchanged, but over the following weeks there was a gradual improvement in power. Postoperative angiography showed the angioma to be obliterated completely. He returned to the referring hospital but was reviewed 6 months later. He was able to get about with 1 stick, was free of pain, had no disturbance of micturition apart from urgency, and was mildly constipated. He had, however, found himself to be impotent.

Comment

The rapidity with which this patient became severely disabled is exemplary. One of the two angiographically-defined arteries feeding the angioma could not be identified within the dura at operation but was found to descend in the extradural tissues to an abnormal knot of vessels related to the other feeder. His somatic and sphincter disturbances improved considerably after operation.

Case 14

Mr D.T., a 44-year-old artisan, was admitted (A 28642) in 1966.

History

Three months before admission he developed numbness in the right thigh, and this spread to the left thigh after 6 weeks and then to the genitalia. 6 weeks before admission his gait became stiff and awkward, and he found he was impotent. A few days later he noticed that he was unable to feel the passage of urine or faeces, and over the following days he developed hesitancy and urgency of micturition, difficulty in appreciating when his bladder was full, and faecal incontinence.

Examination

There was mild spasticity in the legs and a rather variable generalised weakness of the left leg. The ankle jerks and plantar responses were unobtainable. Pin-prick and light touch appreciation were impaired over the sacral dermatomes, especially on the right, and vibration and postural sense were impaired over the lateral three toes of the left foot. His gait was normal.

Investigations

The cerebrospinal fluid contained no cells and a protein concentration of 60 mg per cent. Myelography showed vermiform shadows posterior to the cord below the 9th thoracic vertebral level, without any obstruction to the flow of contrast material. Aortography showed some filling of the malformation but the origin of its blood supply could not be identified; the patient developed flexor and adductor spasms with each injection of contrast material but there was no change in his signs.

Surgery

Laminectomy of the 9th, 10th and 11th thoracic vertebrae was performed and the dura and arachnoid were opened. At the rostral limit of the exposure a small artery ran directly into a large coiled vessel containing partly arterialised blood, which descended the cord in a serpentine manner. Both vessels were divided, as were four small vessels which joined the venous channel as it descended, and the malformation was removed. The laminectomy was then extended to the 1st lumbar vertebra, and the stump of the large venous channel was seen to anastomose with a small artery running up from the tip of the conus, and then to turn toward the anterior surface of the cord. The cord itself was firm but swollen, and some fine vessels ran out on nerve roots from the conus. The abnormal vessels were removed at the limits of the exposure, and the wound was closed in layers.

Subsequent course

He initially showed some improvement in his motor and sphincter disturbances. He decided to return home to Scotland and was followed up at a local hospital. Although his records are no longer available, it seems that about 2 months after operation there was an abrupt increase in his symptoms, which then gradually worsened so that he had to use a frame for walking and suffered occasional urinary incontinence until his death 3 years later.

Comment

It seems reasonable to attribute the deterioration which occurred in this case to an intramedullary component of the angioma since the presence of local cord swelling and of vessels connecting the cord with the extramedullary lesion implies that this was present. It is unlikely to have been due to the operation itself in view of the time course of its development.

Case 15

Mr N.S., a 55-year-old surveyor, was admitted (A 63384) in 1971.

History

He complained of increasing weakness in the legs for 1 year. This commenced 6 weeks after he was involved— but uninjured—in a road traffic accident, and initially affected only the right leg, spreading to the other after about 6 months. His exercise tolerance diminished until eventually he could only walk for about 400 yards with the support of a stick. For 10 months prior to admission he had also had urgency and frequency of micturition, with dysuria and occasional nocturia, and for 4 months he had experienced right sciatic pain which came on with exercise and was relieved by rest. He had been mildly constipated for a few weeks. He was investigated by myelography at his local hospital without a diagnosis being established and was therefore referred to the National Hospital.

Examination

There was slight wasting, gross spasticity, generalised weakness, pathologically brisk tendon reflexes and an extensor plantar response in both legs. All modalities of cutaneous sensation were impaired below the 2nd lumbar dermatome on the left, vibration was not felt below both knees, and postural sense was disturbed in the feet. His gait was spastic.

Investigations

Rescreening of the contrast material which remained in the subarachnoid space from his previous myelograms revealed vermiform defects suggestive of an angioma in the lower thoracic region. Selective spinal angiography showed that the angioma was fed by two vessels which passed through the right 7th and 8th intervertebral foramina and then appeared to unite; they were supplied mainly by the 8th right intercostal artery, but the upper one filled also from the 7th. They ascended to the malformation which was situated posteriorly at the 7th thoracic vertebral level, and large veins descended from it to the lower thoracic region. The artery of Adamkiewicz could not be outlined.

Surgery

After laminectomy of the 7th, 8th and 9th thoracic vertebrae, the dura and arachnoid were opened to reveal a convoluted angioma covering the lower half of the exposed cord. Only one feeding vessel could be identified, and this accompanied the 8th thoracic nerve root; once within the dura it ran straight to the cord and then descended on it, running from side to side. When the artery was clipped the blood within the angioma became darker, although it remained arterialised. The vessel was divided close to the dura, followed caudally and dissected off the cord. It was necessary to perform a partial laminectomy of the 10th thoracic vertebra before the vessel was found to terminate abruptly by running into two thin-walled veins which were divided. The malformation was removed and the dura, muscles and skin were closed.

Subsequent course

His immediate postoperative course was uneventful, but over the course of the following weeks it became apparent that his leg weakness and spasticity were more severe than previously, and he had difficulty in getting about. When last reassessed, 1½ years after leaving hospital, he could walk for only about 200 yards with the support of 2 sticks, and his disturbance of micturition remained unchanged.

Comment

This patient's functional capacity declined immediately after surgery and has since remained unchanged; the deterioration in his condition was probably related, therefore, to the operation itself.

Case 16

Mr H.T., a 58-year-old tax collector, was admitted (65485) in 1968.

History

He complained of increasing weakness of the left arm and leg for 7 months, and of some hesitancy of micturition. He had also noticed occasional twiching of the left thumb which began shortly before the onset of weakness. He gave a past history of recurrent subarachnoid haemorrhage, having had 6 in the preceding 17 years, but carotid and vertebral angiography, performed elsewhere on two occasions, failed to reveal an intracranial source.

Examination

On the left side there was myoclonic jerking of the abductor pollicis brevis muscle, slight wasting of the thenar eminence, mild weakness of grip in the hand, mild spasticity and weakness of the leg, brisk tendon reflexes and an equivocal plantar response. Pin-prick and temperature appreciation were mildly impaired below the 1st thoracic dermatome on the right, and this continued on into the sacral segments but seemed to fade on the leg. Postural sense was reduced in the left toes, and vibration appreciation was impaired in both feet.

Investigations

The cerebrospinal fluid contained less than 1 white cell per cu mm, and a protein concentration of 100 mg per cent. Myelography showed an irregular filling defect and partial obstruction of the flow of contrast material at the level of the 5th and 6th cervical vertebrae, with serpiginous defects extending rostrally and caudally from this region. Bilateral subclavian and vertebral angiography showed that the malformation was located posteriorly at this level and was fed by branches of the deep cervical arteries which entered through the right 5–6 cervical, left 6–7 cervical and right 1–2 thoracic intervertebral foramina. The anterior spinal artery in this region was supplied mainly by the left vertebral artery.

Surgery

Each side of the neck was explored separately, and vessels feeding the malformation were divided extravertebrally.

Subsequent course

He made a good recovery from both operations. Subsequent angiographic studies showed that there was still some filling of a small part of the angioma from the left side, but not from the right. The myoclonic jerking ceased and the limb weakness improved considerably over the following weeks, but he continued to drag his left leg slightly on walking. Five years later he remained well, was leading a full life and complained of no incapacity.

Comment

The spinal source of this patient's recurrent subarachnoid haemorrhage was not recognised until he developed signs of cord dysfunction. As occurs not uncommonly with cervical angiomas, the lesion was fed by several arteries, but their extravertebral occlusion led to a satisfactory outcome in this case.

References

ABBOTT K.H. (1939) Subarachnoid hemorrhage from an ependymoma arising in the filum terminal. Report of a case. *Bulletin of the Los Angeles Neurological Society*, **4**, 127–132.

ADAMKIEWICZ A. (1882) Die Blutgefässe des menschlichen Rückenmarkes. 11. Die Gefässe der Rückenmarkoberfläche. *Sitzungsberichte der Akademie der Wissenschaften in Wien*, **85**, 101–130.

ADAMS H.D. and VAN GEERTRUYDEN H.H. (1956) Neurologic complications of aortic surgery. *Annals of Surgery*, **144**, 574–609.

ALEXANDER W. (1922) Discussion on Angioma racemosum des Rückenmarkes. *Zentralblatt für die gesamte Neurologie und Psychiatrie*, **28**, 246.

AMINOFF M.J., BARNARD R.O. and LOGUE V. (1974) The pathophysiology of spinal vascular malformations. *Journal of the Neurological Sciences*, **23**, 255–263.

AMINOFF M.J. and LOGUE V. (1974a) Clinical features of spinal vascular malformations. *Brain*, **97**, 197–210.

AMINOFF M.J. and LOGUE V. (1974b) The prognosis of patients with spinal vascular malformations. *Brain*, **97**, 211–218.

ANDRÉ-THOMAS, FERRAND, SCHAEFFER and DE MARTEL (1930) Syndrome d'hémorragie méningée réalisé par une tumeur de la queue de cheval. *Paris Médical*, **77**, 292–296.

ANTONI N. (1962) Spinal vascular malformations (angiomas) and myelomalacia. *Neurology* (Minneapolis), **12**, 795–804.

AREY L.B. (1965) *Developmental Anatomy. A textbook and laboratory manual of embryology*, 7th edition. Philadelphia and London: Saunders.

ARSENI C. and SAMITCA D.C. (1959) Vascular malformations of the spinal cord. *Acta psychiatrica et neurologica scandinavica*, **34**, 10–17.

BAILEY W.L. and SPERL M.P. (1969) Angiomas of the cervical spinal cord. *Journal of Neurosurgery*, **30**, 560–568.

BAKER H.L., LOVE J.G. and LAYTON D.D. (1967) Angiographic and surgical aspects of spinal cord vascular anomalies. *Radiology*, **88**, 1078–1085.

BASSETT R.C., PEET M.M. and HOLT J.F. (1949) Pial-medullary angiomas. Clinicopathologic features and treatment. *Archives of Neurology and Psychiatry*, **61**, 558–568.

BÉRAUD R. and MELOCHE B.R. (1965) A propos des malformations vasculaires médullaires. Description de deux cas et revue de littérature. *L'Union Médicale du Canada*, **94**, 176–188.

BERENBRUCH K. (1890) *Ein Fall von Multiplen Angiolipomen Kombiniert mit einem Angiom des Rückenmarks*. Inaugural Dissertation, Tübingen.

BERGSTRAND H. (1936) Die pathologische Anatomie der Hämangiome des Zentralnervensystems. In *Gefässmissbildungen und Gefässegeschwülste des Gehirns* by Bergstrand H., Olivecrona H. and Tonnis W. Pp. 8–68. Leipzig: Thieme.

BERGSTRAND A., HÖÖK O. and LIDVALL H. (1964) Vascular malformations of the spinal cord. *Acta neurologica scandinavica*, **40**, 169–183.

BLACKWOOD W. (1958) Discussion on vascular disease of the spinal cord. *Proceedings of the Royal Society of Medicine*, **51**, 543–547.

BOLTON B. (1939) The blood supply of the human spinal cord. *Journal of Neurology and Psychiatry*, **2**, 137–148.

BRION S., NETSKY M.G. and ZIMMERMAN H.M. (1952) Vascular malformations of the spinal cord. *Archives of Neurology and Psychiatry*, **68**, 339–361.

BUCHANAN D.N. and WALKER A.E. (1941) Vascular anomalies of the spinal cord in children. *American Journal of Diseases of Children*, **61**, 928–932.

CHATTERJEE R.N. (1969) Spinal vascular malformations—their classification, pathogenesis, and the rationale of treatment by excision of the draining veins. *Excerpta Medica*, International Congress Series, No. 193, p. 46.

CHATTERJEE R.N. and ROY R.N. (1968) Spinal vascular malformations and their treatment. *Proceedings of the Australian Association of Neurologists* **5**, 607–610.

COBB S. (1915) Haemangioma of the spinal cord associated with skin naevi of the same metamere. *Annals of Surgery*, **62**, 641–649.

CRAIGIE E.H. (1972) Vascular supply of the spinal cord. In *The Spinal Cord. Basic Aspects and Surgical Considerations*, edited by Austin G. Pp. 59–87. Springfield: Thomas.

CROSS G.O. (1947) Subarachnoid cervical angioma with cutaneous hemangioma of a corresponding metamere. *Archives of Neurology and Psychiatry*, **58**, 359–366.

CUSHING H. and BAILEY P. (1928) *Tumors arising from the bloodvessels of the brain.* Springfield, Illinois: Thomas.

DELMAS-MARSALET P. (1941) Poussées évolutives gravidiques et image lipiodolée caractéristiques des hémangiomes médullaires. *Press Médicale*, **49**, 964–965.

DEN HARTOG JAGER W.A. (1949) About two new forms in the group of the phacomatoses. *Folia psychiatrica, neurologica et neurochirurgica neerlandica*, **52**, 356–364.

DI CHIRO G. (1957) Combined retino-cerebellar angiomatosis and deep cervical angiomas. *Journal of Neurosurgery*, **14**, 685–687.

DI CHIRO G. (1972) Recent successes and failures in radiographic and radioisotopic angiography of the spinal cord. *British Journal of Radiology*, **45**, 553–560.

DI CHIRO G., DOPPMAN J.L., and OMMAYA A.K. (1967) Selective arteriography of arteriovenous aneurysms of the spinal cord. *Radiology*, **88**, 1065–1077.

DI CHIRO G., JONES A.E., JOHNSTON G.S. and ALLEN F.H. (1973) Value and limits of radionuclide angiography of the spinal cord. *Radiology*, **109**, 125–130.

DI CHIRO G. and WENER L. (1973) Angiography of the spinal cord. A review of contemporary techniques and applications. *Journal of Neurosurgery*, **39**, 1–29.

DILENGE D., HÉON M. and METZGER J. (1973) Selective spinal angiography in multiple CNS lesions. *Journal de l'Association Canadienne des Radiologistes*, **24**, 178–183.

DJINDJIAN R. (1972) Neuroradiological examination of spinal cord angiomas. In *Handbook of Clinical Neurology* Volume 12, pp. 631–643, edited by Vinken P.J. and Bruyn G.W. Amsterdam: North-Holland.

DJINDJIAN R., COPHIGNON J., REY A., THÉRON J., MERLAND J.J. and HOUDART R. (1973) Superselective arteriographic embolization by the femoral route in neuroradiology. Study of 50 cases. 11. Embolization in vertebromedullary pathology. *Neuroradiology* **6**, 132–142.

DJINDJIAN R., HOUDART R. and HURTH M. (1969) *Les angiomes de la moelle.* Paris: Editions Sandoz.

DJINDJIAN R., HURTH M. and HOUDART R. (1970) *L'Angiographie de la moelle épinière.* Paris: Masson.

DOPPMAN J.L. and DI CHIRO G. (1965) Subtraction-angiography of spinal cord vascular malformations. Report of a case. *Journal of Neurosurgery*, **23**, 440–443.

DOPPMAN J.L., DI CHIRO G. and OMMAYA A. (1968) Obliteration of spinal-cord arteriovenous malformation by percutaneous embolisation. *Lancet*, **1**, 477.

DOPPMAN J.L., DI CHIRO G. and OMMAYA A.K. (1969) *Selective arteriography of the spinal cord.* St. Louis: Green.

170 *References*

DOPPMAN J.L., DI CHIRO G. and OMMAYA A.K. (1971) Percutaneous embolization of spinal cord arteriovenous malformations. *Journal of Neurosurgery*, **34**, 48–55.

DOPPMAN J.L., WIRTH F.P., DI CHIRO G. and OMMAYA A.K. (1969) Value of cutaneous angiomas in the arteriographic localization of spinal-cord arteriovenous malformations. *New England Journal of Medicine*, **281**, 1440–1444.

DOUGLAS-WILSON H., MILLER S. and WATSON G.W. (1933) Spontaneous subarachnoid haemorrhage of intraspinal origin. *British Medical Journal*, **1**, 554–555.

ECHOLS D.H. and HOLCOMBE R.G. (1940–1) Extramedullary aneurysm of the spinal cord. *New Orleans Medical and Surgical Journal*, **93**, 582–583.

ELSBERG C.A. (1916) The surgical significance and operative treatment of enlarged and varicose veins of the spinal cord. *American Journal of the Medical Sciences*, **61**, 642–652.

EPSTEIN J.A., BELLER A.J. and COHEN I. (1949) Arterial anomalies of the spinal cord. *Journal of Neurosurgery*, **6**, 45–56.

FAZIO G. (1939) L'angioarchitettonica del midollo spinale umano e i suoi rapporti con le cito-mielo-architettonica. *Rivista di Patologia nervosa e mentale*, **52**, 252–291.

FINCHER E.F. (1951) Spontaneous subarachnoid hemorrhage in intradural tumors of the lumbar sac. A clinical syndrome. *Journal of Neurosurgery*, **8**, 576–584.

FINE R.D. (1961) Angioma racemosum venosum of spinal cord with segmentally related angiomatous lesions of skin and forearm. *Journal of Neurosurgery*, **18**, 546–550.

FOIX CH. and ALAJOUANINE TH. (1926) La myelite necrotique subaigue. *Revue neurologique*, **33**, ii, 1–42.

FORD F.R. (1944) *Diseases of the Nervous System in Infancy, Childhood and Adolescence.* 2nd edition. Springfield, Illinois: Thomas.

FRIED L.C., DI CHIRO G. and DOPPMAN J.L. (1969) Ligation of major thoraco-lumbar spinal cord arteries in monkeys. *Journal of Neurosurgery*, **31**, 608–614.

GAUPP J. (1888) Casuistische Beiträge zur pathologischen Anatomie des Rückenmarks und siner Häute. *Beiträge zur pathologischen Anatomie und Physiologie*, **2**, 510–524.

GAUTIER-SMITH P.C. (1967) Clinical aspects of spinal neurofibromas. *Brain*, **90**, 359–394.

GILBERT I. (1952) Angioma venosum racemosum with angiomatous lesions of skin and omentum. *British Medical Journal*, **1**, 468–470.

GILLILAN L.A. (1958) The arterial blood supply of the human spinal cord. *Journal of Comparative Neurology*, **110**, 75–103.

GILLILAN L.A. (1970) Veins of the spinal cord. *Neurology* (Minneapolis), **20**, 860–868.

GIRARD P.-F. and GARDE A. (1955) Les angiomes de la moelle (angiomes racemeux veineux et a court-circuit arterio-veineux). *Gazette médicale de France*, **62**, 1175–1185.

GROSS S.W. and RALSTON B.L. (1959) Vascular malformations of the spinal cord. *Surgery, Gynecology and Obstetrics*, **108**, 673–678.

GUILLAIN G. and ALAJOUANINE T. (1925) Paraplégie par compression due à un volumineux angiocèle de la pie-mère spinale. Contribution à l'étude des compressions médullaires dues à des formations vasculaires pathologiques. *Journal de Neurologie et de Psychiatrie*, Bruxelles, **25**, 689–698.

References 171

HALPERN L., FELDMAN S. and PEYSER E. (1958) Subarachnoid hemorrhage with papilledema due to spinal neurofibroma. *Archives of Neurology and Psychiatry*, **79**, 138–141.

HAMBY W.B. (1948) Spontaneous subarachnoid hemorrhage of aneurysmal origin. Factors influencing prognosis. *Journal of the American Medical Association*, **136**, 522–527.

HAMILTON W.J. and MOSSMAN H.W. (1972) *Hamilton, Boyd and Mossman's Human Embryology*. 4th edition. Cambridge: Heffer.

HENSON R.A. and CROFT P.B. (1956) Spontaneous spinal subarachnoid haemorrhage. *Quarterly Journal of Medicine*, **25**, 53–66.

HERDT J.R., DI CHIRO G. and DOPPMAN J.L. (1971) Combined arterial and arteriovenous aneurysms of the spinal cord. *Radiology*, **99**, 589–593.

HERREN R.Y. and ALEXANDER L. (1939) Sulcal and intrinsic blood vessels of human spinal cord. *Archives of Neurology and Psychiatry*, **41**, 678–687.

HÖÖK O. and LIDVALL H. (1958) Arteriovenous aneurysms of the spinal cord. A report of two cases investigated by vertebral angiography. *Journal of Neurosurgery*, **15**, 84–91.

HOUDART R. and DJINDJIAN R. (1966) Angiomas of the spinal cord. *Proceedings of the Royal Society of Medicine*, **59**, 787–790.

HOUDART R., DJINDJIAN R. and HURTH M. (1966) Vascular malformations of the spinal cord. *Journal of Neurosurgery*, **24**, 583–594.

JACKSON F. and HUSSEY M. (1967) Spinal extramedullary arteriovenous fistula: successful removal with reversal of neurological signs following failure of initial decompressive laminectomy. *Military Medicine*, **132**, 22–24.

JELLINGER K. and NEUMAYER E. (1972) Claudication of the spinal cord and cauda equina. In *Handbook of Clinical Neurology*, volume 12, pp. 507–547. Edited by Vinken P.J. and Bruyn G.W. Amsterdam: North-Holland.

KADYI H. (1889) *Über die Blutgefässe des menschlichen Rückenmarkes*. Lemberg: Gubrynowicz and Schmidt.

KAPLAN G., ROSWIT B. and KRUEGER E.G. (1952) Results of radiation therapy in vascular anomalies of the central nervous system. *Radiology*, **59**, 555–558.

KAUFMAN H.H., OMMAYA A.K., DI CHIRO G. and DOPPMAN J.L. (1970) Compression vs "steal". The pathogenesis of symptoms in arterio-venous malformations of the spinal cord. *Archives of Neurology*, **23**, 173–178.

KISSEL P. and DUREUX J.B. (1972) Cobb syndrome. Cutaneomeningospinal angiomatosis. In *Handbook of Clinical Neurology*, volume 12, pp. 429–445. Edited by Vinken P.J. and Bruyn G.W. Amsterdam: North-Holland.

KRAYENBÜHL H. (1947) Spontane spinal Subarachnoidalblutung und akute Rückenmarkskompression bei intraduralem, spinalem Neurinom. *Schweizerische Medizinische Wochenschrift*, **77**, 692–694.

KRAYENBÜHL H. and YAŞARGIL M.G. (1963) Die Varicosis spinalis und ihre Behandlung. *Schweizer Archiv für Neurologie und Psychiatrie*, **92**, 74–92.

KRAYENBÜHL H., YAŞARGIL M.G. and McCLINTOCK H.G. (1969) Treatment of spinal cord vascular malformations by surgical excision. *Journal of Neurosurgery*, **30**, 427–435.

KRENCHEL N.J. (1961) *Intracranial racemose angiomas. A clinical study*. Aarhus: Universitetsforlaget.

KRIEGER A.J. (1972) A vascular malformation of the spinal cord in association with a cauda equina ependymoma. *Vascular Surgery*, **6**, 167–172.

KRISHNAN K.R. and SMITH W.T. (1961) Intramedullary haemangioblastoma of the spinal cord associated with pial varicosities simulating intradural angioma. *Journal of Neurology, Neurosurgery, and Psychiatry*, **24**, 350–352.

KUNC Z. and BRET J. (1969) Diagnosis and treatment of vascular malformations of the spinal cord. *Journal of Neurosurgery*, **30**, 436–445.

LAZORTHES G. (1972) Pathology, classification and clinical aspects of vascular diseases of the spinal cord. In *Handbook of Clinical Neurology*, volume 12, pp. 492–506, edited by Vinken P.J. and Bruyn G.W. Amsterdam: North-Holland.

LAZORTHES G. and GOUAZÉ A. (1968) Cited by Lazorthes G. (1972).

LAZORTHES G., GOUAZÉ A., BASTIDE G., SANTINI J.J., ZADEH O. and BURDIN PH. (1966) La vascularisation artérielle de la moelle cervicale. Étude des suppléances. *Revue neurologique*, **115**, 1055–1068.

LAZORTHES G., GOUAZÉ A., BASTIDE G., SOUTOUL J.-H., ZADEH O. and SANTINI J.-J. (1966) La vascularisation artérielle du renflement lombaire; étude des variations et des suppléances. *Revue neurologique*, **114**, 109–122.

LAZORTHES G., POULHES J., BASTIDE G., ROULLEAU J. and CHANCHOLLE A.-R. (1958) La vascularisation artérielle de la moelle. Recherches anatomiques et applications à la pathologie medullaire et à la pathologie aortique. *Neurochirurgie*, **4**, 3–19.

LOCKSLEY H.B. (1966) Report on the cooperative study of intracranial aneurysms and subarachnoid hemorrhage, Section V, Part 11. Natural history of subarachnoid hemorrhage, intracranial aneurysms and arteriovenous malformations. *Journal of Neurosurgery*, **25**, 321–368.

LOGUE V., AMINOFF M.J. and KENDALL B.E. (1974) Results of surgical treatment for patients with a spinal angioma. *Journal of Neurology, Neurosurgery, and Psychiatry*. **37**, 1074–1081.

LOMBARDI G. and MIGLIAVACCA F. (1959) Angiomas of the spinal cord. *British Journal of Radiology*, **32**, 810–814.

LUESSENHOP A.J. and DELA CRUZ T. (1969) The surgical excision of spinal intradural vascular malformations. *Journal of Neurosurgery*, **30**, 552–559.

MCALPINE D. and COMPSTON N. (1952) Some aspects of the natural history of disseminated sclerosis. *Quarterly Journal of Medicine*, **21**, 135–167.

MATTHEWS W.B. (1959) The spinal bruit. *Lancet*, **2**, 1117–1118.

MICHAEL J.C. and LEVIN P.M. (1936) Multiple telangiectases of the brain. *Archives of Neurology and Psychiatry*, **36**, 514–529.

MORRIS L. (1960) Angioma of the cervical spinal cord. *Radiology*, **75**, 785–787.

MURRAY P.D.F. (1928) Chorio-allantoic grafts of fragments of the two-day chick, with special reference to the development of the limbs, intestine, and skin. *Australian Journal of Experimental Biology and Medical Science*, **5**, 237–256.

NEWMAN M.J.D. (1958) Spinal angioma with symptoms in pregnancy. *Journal of Neurology, Neurosurgery, and Psychiatry*, **21**, 38–41.

NEWMAN M.J.D. (1959) Racemose angioma of the spinal cord. *Quarterly Journal of Medicine*, **28**, 97–108.

References 173

NEWQUIST R.E. and MAYFIELD F.H. (1960) Spinal angioma presenting during pregnancy. *Journal of Neurosurgery*, **17**, 541–545.
NEWTON T.H. and ADAMS J.E. (1968) Angiographic demonstration and non-surgical embolization of spinal cord angioma. *Radiology*, **91**, 873–876.
NIELSEN J.M., MARVIN S.L. and SELETZ E. (1958) Telangiectasis of skin and spinal cord. *Bulletin of the Los Angeles Neurological Society*, **23**, 97–101.

ODOM G.L. (1962) Vascular lesions of the spinal cord: malformations, spinal subarachnoid and extradural hemorrhage. *Clinical Neurosurgery*, **8**, 196–236.
ODOM G.L., WOODHALL B. and MARGOLIS G. (1957) Spontaneous hematomyelia and angiomas of the spinal cord. *Journal of Neurosurgery*, **14**, 192–202.
OLIVECRONA H. and LADENHEIM J. (1957) *Congenital arteriovenous aneurysms of the carotid and vertebral arterial systems*. Berlin: Springer-Verlag.
OMMAYA A.K., DI CHIRO G. and DOPPMAN J. (1969) Ligation of arterial supply in the treatment of spinal cord arteriovenous malformations. *Journal of Neurosurgery*, **30**, 679–692.

PADGET D.H. (1954) Designation of the embryonic intersegmental arteries in reference to the vertebral artery and subclavian stem. *Anatomical Record*, **119**, 349–356.
PIA H.W. (1973) Diagnosis and treatment of spinal angiomas. *Acta Neurochirurgica*, **28**, 1–12.
PIA H.W. and VOGELSANG H. (1965) Diagnose und therapie spinaler angiome. *Deutsche Zeitschrift für Nervenheilkunde*, **187**, 74–96.
PAPPENHEIM E. (1938) Angioma racemosum des Cervicalmarks und Hämatomyelie. *Deutsche Zeitschrift für Nervenheilkinde*, **146**, 284–293.
POUYANNE L., BERGOUIGNAN M. and CAILLON F. (1950) Angiomes racèmeux de la moelle. *Revue neurologique*, **83**, 494–497.
PRIETO A. and CANTU R.C. (1967) Spinal subarachnoid hemorrhage associated with neurofibroma of the cauda equina. *Journal of Neurosurgery*, **27**, 63–69.

RAND C.W. (1927) Hemangioma of the spinal cord. *Archives of Neurology and Psychiatry*, **18**, 755–765.
RANSOME G.A. and MEKIE E.C. (1942) A varix of the spinal cord. Case report with a diagnostic radiological appearance and description of tumour. *British Journal of Surgery*, **29**, 330–335.
RASMINSKY M. (1973) The effects of temperature on conduction in demyelinated single nerve fibers. *Archives of Neurology*, **28**, 287–292.
ROGER H., PAILLAS J.-E., BONNAL J. and VIGOUROUX R. (1951) Angiomes de la moelle et des racines. *Acta neurologica et psychiatrica belgica*, **51**, 491–495.
ROGER H., PAILLAS J.-E. and DUPLAY J. (1949) Hémorragie méningée spino-cérebrale révélatrice d'une tumeur de la queue de cheval chez deux jeunes sujets. *Bulletins et memoires de la Société médicale des Hopitaux de Paris*, **65**, 37–40.
RUSSELL D.S. and RUBINSTEIN L.J. (1959) *Pathology of tumours of the nervous system*. London: Arnold.

SARGENT P. (1925) Haemangeioma of the pia mater causing compression paraplegia. *Brain*, **48**, 259–267.
SCHOTT B., COTTE L., TRILLET M. and BADY B. (1963) Sémiologie "encéphalique" des hémorragies méningées spinales. (A

174 *References*

propos de 2 observations de malformations vasculaires de la moelle.) *Revue neurologique*, **109**, 654–657.

SCOVILLE W.B. (1948) Intramedullary arteriovenous aneurysm of the spinal cord. *Journal of Neurosurgery*, **5**, 307–312.

SHAPIRO R. (1968) *Myelography.* Chicago: Year Book Medical Publishers. 2nd edition.

SHEPHARD R.H. (1963) Observations on intradural spinal angioma: treatment by excision. *Neurochirurgia* (Stuttgart), **6**, 58–74.

SHEPHARD R.H. (1965) Some new concepts in intradural spinal angioma. *Rivista di Patologia nervosa e mentale*, **86**, 276–283.

STEIN S.C., OMMAYA A.K., DOPPMAN J.L. and DI CHIRO G. (1972) Arteriovenous malformation of the cauda equina with arterial supply from branches of the internal iliac arteries. *Journal of Neurosurgery*, **36**, 649–651.

STERLING WL. and JAKIMOWICZ WL. (1936) Rozstrzenie żylne opon miekkich rdzenia i naczyniakowatość śródrdzeniowa. *Neurologja Polska*, **19**, 391–408.

STRAIN R.E. (1964) Surgical treatment of angiomas of the spinal cord. *American Surgeon*, **30**, 163–166.

SUH T.H. and ALEXANDER L. (1939) Vascular system of the human spinal cord. *Archives of Neurology and Psychiatry*, **41**, 659–677.

Szojchet A. (1968) Metameric spinal cord and skin hemangiomas. Case report. *Journal of Neurosurgery*, **29**, 199–201.

TARLOV I.M. and KEENER E.B. (1953) Subarachnoid hemorrhage and tumor implants from spinal sarcoma in an infant. *Neurology* (Minneapolis), **3**, 384–390.

TENG P. and PAPATHEODOROU C. (1964) Myelographic appearance of vascular anomalies of the spinal cord. *British Journal of Radiology*, **37**, 358–366.

TENG P. and SHAPIRO M.J. (1958) Arterial anomalies of the spinal cord. Myelographic diagnosis and treatment by section of dentate ligaments. *Archives of Neurology and Psychiatry*, **80**, 577–586.

THERKELSEN J. (1958) Angioma racemosum venosum medullae spinalis. *Acta psychiatrica et neurologica scandinavica*, **33**, 219–231.

TORR, J.B.D. (1957) The embryological development of the anterior spinal artery in man. *Journal of Anatomy*, **91**, 587.

TRUPP M. and SACHS E. (1948) Vascular tumors of the brain and spinal cord and their treatment. *Journal of Neurosurgery*, **5**, 354–371.

TUREEN L.L. (1938) Circulation of the spinal cord and the effect of vascular occlusion. *Association for Research into Nervous and Mental Disease. Research Publications*, **18**, 394–437.

TURNBULL I.M. (1972) Blood supply of the spinal cord. In *Handbook of Clinical Neurology*, volume 12, pp. 478–491, edited by Vinken P.J. and Bruyn G.W. Amsterdam: North-Holland.

TURNER O.A. and KERNOHAN J.W. (1941) Vascular malformations and vascular tumors involving the spinal cord. A pathologic study of forty-six cases. *Archives of Neurology and Psychiatry*, **46**, 444–463.

VAN BOGAERT L. (1950) Pathologie des angiomatoses. *Acta neurologica et psychiatrica belgica*, **50**, 525–610.

VERBIEST H. and CALLIAUW L. (1960) Les angiomes racémeux intraduraux de la moelle épinière. *Revue neurologique*, **102**, 230–243.

VRAA-JENSEN G. (1949) Angioma of the spinal cord. *Acta psychiatrica et neurologica scandinavica*, **24**, 709–721.

WALTON J.N. (1953) Subarachnoid haemorrhage of unusual aetiology. *Neurology* (Minneapolis), **3**, 517–543.
WALTON J.N. (1956) *Subarachnoid Haemorrhage*. Edinburgh and London: Livingstone.
WILSON S.A.K. (1955) *Neurology*, 2nd edition, edited by Bruce A.N. London: Butterworth.
WIRTH F.P., POST K.D., DI CHIRO G., DOPPMAN J.L. and OMMAYA A.K. (1970) Foix-Alajouanine disease. Spontaneous thrombosis of a spinal cord arteriovenous malformation: a case report. *Neurology* (Minneapolis), **20**, 1114–1118.
WYBURN-MASON R. (1943) *The vascular abnormalities and tumours of the spinal cord and its membranes*. London: Kimpton.

YUHL E.T. (1955) Spontaneous intraspinal hemorrhage and paraplegia complicating bishydroxycoumarin (Dicumarol) therapy. *Archives of Neurology and Psychiatry*, **73**, 570–572.

Index